# THE EAR BOOK

# THE EAR BOOK

## A PARENT'S GUIDE TO COMMON EAR DISORDERS OF CHILDREN

*DAVID R. MARTY, M.D.*

Lang E.N.T. Publishing, Jefferson City, Missouri

THE EAR BOOK

A PARENT'S GUIDE TO COMMON EAR DISORDERS OF CHILDREN

David R. Marty, M.D.

The information contained in this book is based upon the knowledge and experience of the author at the time of publication. It has been reviewed for accuracy by other medical doctors. The author, publisher and reviewers disclaim all responsibility arising from any adverse effects or results which occur or might occur as a result of the use of any of the information contained in the book. If you have any question or concern about the appropriateness or application of the information described in this book, consult your physician.

Published by:

Lang E.N.T. Publishing
Post Office Box 6846
Jefferson City, MO 65101, U.S.A.
(314) 893-5545


First Printing 1987
Printed in the United States of America

**Library of Congress Cataloging-in-Publication-Data:**

Marty, David R., 1948-
The ear book.

Includes index.
1. Children—Diseases. 2. Ear—Diseases. 3. Ear—Care and hygiene. I. Title. [DNLM: Ear Diseases—in infancy & childhood—popular works. WV 200 M388e]
RF122.5.C4M37 1987 617.8'088054 87-16993
ISBN 0-943023-11-4 (lib. bdg.)
ISBN 0-943023-12-2 (soft)

# DEDICATION

To Lynn, David, Elizabeth and Eric

# FOREWORD

by
Tom Ferguson, M.D.

We are in the early stages of an important medical revolution: We are moving *away* from an old, physician-centered health care system, in which the physician did everything and the client or patient did nothing. We are moving *toward* a new, self-care-based health care system in which laypeople will be encouraged to learn important medical skills, keep up to date on the latest health information, and to take a much greater degree of responsibility for their own health care — and that of their family.

Dr. David Marty's *The Ear Book* is an important part of this self-care revolution. Childhood ear infections are one of the most common health problems in children. Learning to do an ear examination on your child is an excellent way for health-responsible parents to take more control of their family's health. As a physician, an ear specialist, a father, and a long-time self-care advocate, David Marty is uniquely equipped to guide the concerned parent through the steps of learning this important physical examination skill.

As Dr. Marty points out, there are distinct medical advantages of having a family member as part of the health care team. But there are long-term benefits as well: Children who see their parents mastering basic medical skills and taking a high degree of health responsibility will grow up believing that they can do likewise. Thus in addition to helping the motivated parent keep their children healthier, *The Ear Book* will also help set the foundation for raising health-responsible children.

— Tom Ferguson, M.D.
Editor-in-Chief
*Medical Self-Care* Magazine

# ACKNOWLEDGEMENTS

My thanks to the many people who have contributed to the publication of this book, including:

Lew Nash, Marge Cunningham, Suzette Heiman, William Davis, M.D., Lee Rea, M.D., Jane Bell, Tom Ferguson, M.D., Keith Sehnert, M.D. and the many parents who have been so inspiring, especially Joyce and Jerry Kraus and Jean and Russell Marty.

This book would not have been possible without the color photographs provided by Michael Hawke, M.D., Toronto, Canada.

COVER DESIGN: Bill and Gigi Schrader
COVER PHOTOGRAPHY: Zeal Wright
ARTWORK: Kristy Morris
PRINTED BY: The Ovid Bell Press, Inc., Fulton, Mo.

# INTRODUCTION

Interest in self-diagnosis and self-care will be a major trend in health care in the next decade. Patients are demanding more availalble care of the highest quality and at the lowest cost. They are questioning the doctor. They want to participate. They should.

A glance at any bookstore's Health Section will attest to these statements. There are scores of diet books, baby books, exercise books, anatomy books — the list goes on and on. There are, however, no books about one of the most common of all problems, ear disorders of childhood. Many hypertensive patients have their own blood pressure cuffs and stethoscopes, but how many parents are able to examine their own child's ear in the middle of the night? Even if parents are able to purchase an otoscope through their physician, can the examination be performed safely and the findings interpreted accurately? Do the parents know when home care is appropriate and when to call their doctor?

With this book and an otoscope (see ordering information at the back of the book) parents can finally begin to take an active role in the management of their children's ear problems, safely, effectively and at any time of the day or night.

There is no doubt that it is dangerous for parents (myself included) to assume total responsibility for their child's health care. Parents are, however, obligated to recognize and understand common disorders, and to know when to call for help. This book is designed to bridge the communication gap which often occurs between parents and physicians. It is not designed to replace the doctor, but to make parents more effective participants in their family's health care.

It is impossible to discuss all of the various ear diseases. It is also impossible to touch upon all medical conditions which may have symptoms and findings related to the ears. Furthermore, even the "experts" sometimes disagree on diagnosis and management of illnesses. For these reasons, only the common ear disorders are discussed.

# HOW TO USE THIS BOOK

This book has several purposes. The first purpose is to familiarize you with the common ear disorders of children. Second, it is designed to assist you in the recognition of these conditions by showing you how to use an otoscope. Third, you will learn when home care is appropriate and when you should consult your doctor. To reach these goals, the book must be used properly. Don't let it gather dust until 2 a.m. when the ear infection starts.

A diagnosis is really just an educated guess; a very educated, and a very important guess. The more facts you have, the more accurate the "guess" is going to be. Facts are gathered by noting the history of the illness and by observing the patient. These are the symptoms and the signs of an illness. By comparing the symptoms and findings with those of known illnesses, you arrive at a diagnosis. In order to do this, you must first understand the structure (anatomy) and functioning (physiology) of the ears. It is imperative that these sections of the book be mastered first. Then, and only then does the book become useful. Familiarize yourself with the entire book before you need to use it "for real." Concentrate on the first few problems in chapters four, five and six. These are the ones you are most likely to encounter.

This is a problem-oriented book. You must first identify a problem (usually a symptom or complaint) and then find that problem in the book. If you don't find it, you need help from your doctor. There are chapters on ear care, ear pain, ear drainage and hearing loss. Each chapter, in turn, lists a table of contents of the common conditions to be discussed which can cause that specific problem (the most frequently occurring problems are discussed first). Each condition is presented with a general discussion and a capsule summary for review and reference. Where useful, the conditions are also illustrated with a "typical case history." Taking the review tests at the end of each chapter is a good way to make sure you understand the information. Cross references are provided for your convenience; use them when you come to them.

Next comes the fun part: PRACTICE. You will benefit from a spouse or friend with whom you can study and practice regularly. Pretend to have an illness and make your study partner guess it in 10 questions or less. Perhaps you could form a neighborhood study group. You may need a second opinion sometime! Quiz each other and examine each other. Examine your kids and your neighbor's children when they are well (with permission of course). How can you recognize abnormalities if you don't know what a normal ear looks like? You will find there are many variations of "normal." Practice and review if you want to become proficient.

When using the book "for real," you will do just fine if you have done your homework. This book is not the final word on ear disorders, it is only a guide. If there is a question about the information in the book or its application to the problem at hand, contact your physician.

# TABLE OF CONTENTS

# 1

# ANATOMY AND PHYSIOLOGY OF THE EAR

# 1 ANATOMY AND PHYSIOLOGY OF THE EAR

In this section you will learn:

1. The parts of the external, middle and inner ear.
2. How sound is transferred through the ear to the brain.
3. Where hearing loss can occur.
4. The middle ear is the most common site of childhood ear diseases.

Any understanding of illness must be based upon a knowledge of normal structure (anatomy) and function (physiology). In presenting the basics, I will do my best to keep it simple, while offering the appropriate medical terms for those who wish to learn them.

The anatomy of the ear is best considered in three parts: the external ear (the outer ear and canal), the middle ear (the eardrum, middle ear space, middle ear bones, mastoid and Eustachian tube) and the inner ear (the hearing organ and balance organ).

## *THE EXTERNAL EAR*

The external ear consists of the ear itself (pinna or auricle) and the external ear canal down to the eardrum. The important feature about the external ear is that it is composed of a cartilage framework covered by skin. Contrary to popular belief, the pinna does not significantly amplify incoming sounds.

The ear canal varies in length from less than one half inch in newborns to about an inch and one half in adults. Curving downward and forward, it ends at the eardrum (tympanic membrane) which is part

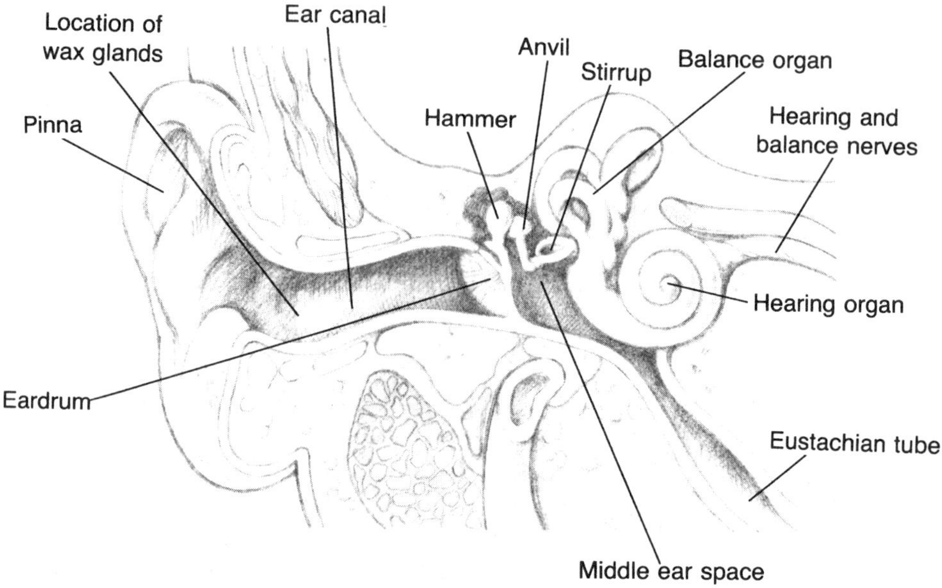


*FIGURE 1*
*Anatomy of the Right Ear Seen from the Front*

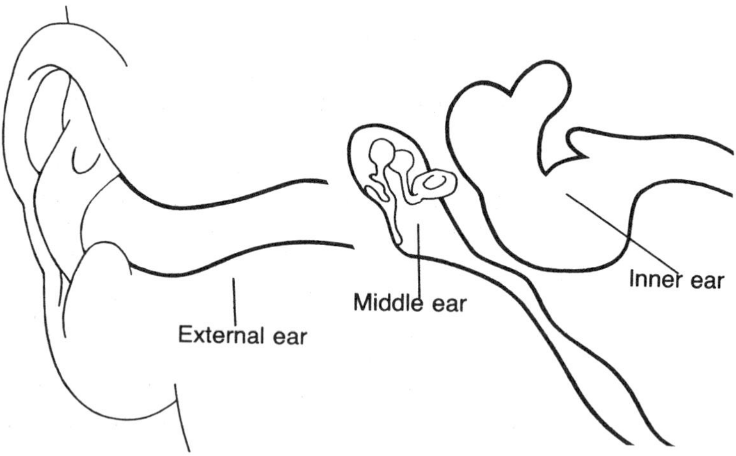

of the middle ear. Protective ear wax (cerumen) of various color, consistency and amount is produced by wax glands in the outer part of the canal. See figure 1.

## *THE MIDDLE EAR*

The middle ear is the site of most ear disease in children and is therefore deserving of special attention. It consists of the eardrum, the middle ear space, the tiny middle ear bones (ossicles) and the passageway leading to the back of the nose (Eustachian tube). Continuous with the middle ear space is a honey-combed network of air pockets in the bone behind the ear, the mastoid. Let's look at each of these parts of the middle ear system.

Separating the ear canal from the middle ear space is a delicate, thin membrane called the eardrum or tympanic membrane. It is paper-thin, semitransparent (like wax paper) and gives you the correct impression that you can almost see through it. It is a three-layered structure, the middle layer of which gives it support and provides attachment to the ear canal. The drum is cone-shaped and slightly tilted, so that the upper part of it is nearer the outside than the rest of it. This characteristic shape causes a glare of light to be seen in the lower, front part of the eardrum when it is viewed through an otoscope, the instrument with which the ear is examined. (Later, you will learn how to safely and properly use it, too.)

The middle ear bones are suspended between the eardrum and the inner ear hearing organ in the middle ear space. Attached to the drum and easily seen through the otoscope is a portion of the hammer (malleus). At a deeper level, parts of the anvil (incus) and stirrup (stapes) are sometimes hazily seen behind the upper, back part of the eardrum. See figures 1 and 2.

The passageway which connects the middle ear space to the nose is called the Eustachian tube. In children, it is shorter in length, and more horizontal. This presumably allows easy access of nasal and throat bacteria to the middle ear, resulting in a greater number of ear infections in children than in adults.

The middle ear connects directly to the mastoid system of air pockets which make up the bony prominence behind the ear. The nerve which supplies the muscles of the face travels through the middle ear and mastoid to exit below the ear. Because of its closeness to the middle ear, facial paralysis is sometimes seen as a complication of ear disease. The nerve is functioning properly when one is able to close the eyes, wrinkle the forehead and purse the lips.

The function of the middle ear system is to amplify and direct sound vibrations into the hearing organ where they are converted into electrical energy and sent on to the brain for interpretation. To allow maximum vibration of the eardrum, there must be air behind it (in the middle ear space) that is equal in pressure to the atmospheric air on the outside of the drum. Otherwise, the eardrum would either be pushed out or pulled in slightly and proper vibration could not occur. This tightening of the drum from pressure differences between the inside and outside results in a sensation of fullness that we all have experienced at times. Proper pressure maintainance is the function of the Eustachian tube, which opens and closes with yawning, chewing and swallowing. As will be seen later, blockage or malfunctioning of the Eustachian tube may lead to ear disease. See figure 1.

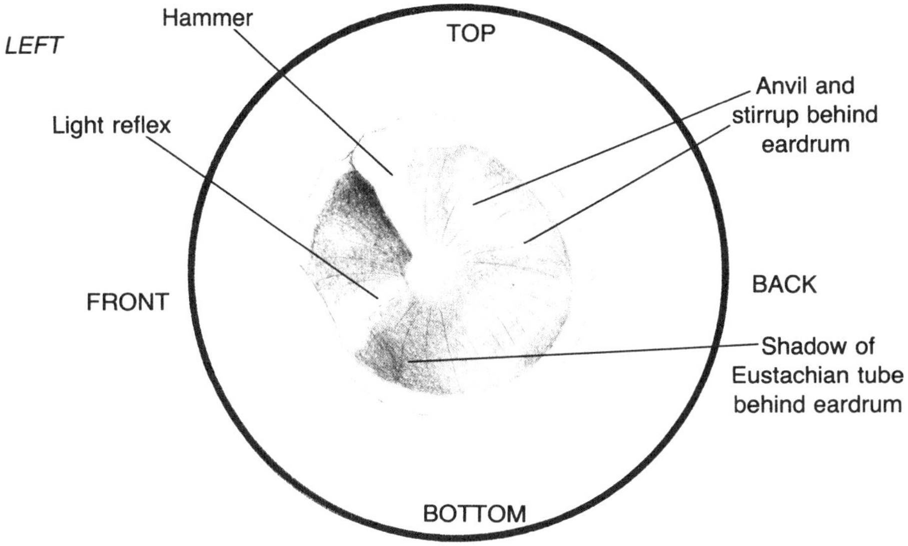


*FIGURE 2*

*Anatomy of the Left and Right Eardrums*
*Seen with an Otoscope*
*(see color plate #1)*

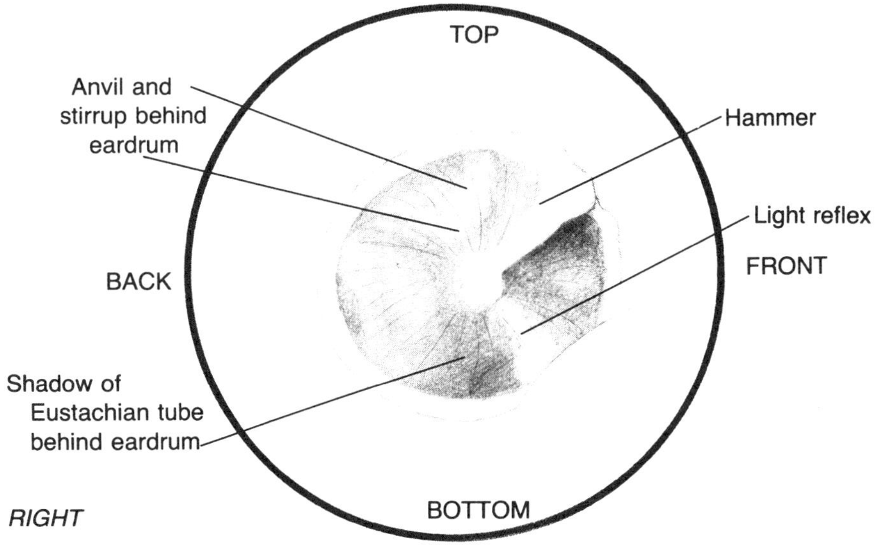

## THE INNER EAR

The inner ear is by far the least understood and most complicated part of the entire ear, but fortunately is rarely the site of childhood illness. It has two components, the hearing organ (cochlea) and the balance organ (vestibular organ). A detailed account of the anatomy and physiology of the inner ear is beyond the scope of this book but a basic understanding is important.

Both organs are capable of converting mechanical energy into electrical signals which are then transmitted to the brain along the hearing and balance nerves. Hearing losses originating in the inner ear are best thought of as electrical problems and are called "sensorineural" hearing losses. (Hearing losses originating in the middle ear structures are mechanical in nature and are called "conductive" hearing losses.) As will be seen in the section on hearing testing (audiometry) the site and amount of hearing loss can usually be determined.

Because the balance organ is near the hearing organ and middle ear, it is sometimes involved in diseases, resulting in the symptom of spinning dizziness (vertigo). The function of the balance organ is to interpret movements of the head and send this information to the brain for correlation with information being received from the eyes, and various muscles of the body. Without the proper functioning of all systems, the sense of balance is disturbed. The beauty and poise of ice-skaters, tennis players and tightrope artists testifies to the amazing job the vestibular organ must do.

## *FOR REVIEW*

I. Match the structures with their location in the ear:

| | |
|---|---|
| 1. Hearing organ | A. External ear |
| 2. Wax glands | B. Middle ear |
| 3. Hammer | C. Inner ear |
| 4. Eustachian tube | |
| 5. Pinna | |
| 6. Vestibular organ | |
| 7. Eardrum | |
| 8. Mastoid | |

II. True or False

9. The function of the external ear is to amplify sounds
10. Soundwaves pass from the stirrup to the eardrum.
11. A problem in the hearing organ might cause an electrical (sensorineural) hearing loss.
12. A sensation of fullness in the ear which occurs during air travel results from middle ear pressure not being equalized through the Eustachian tube.
13. Most ear problems in children occur in the external canal.
14. All dizziness results from inner ear disease.
15. Keeping the right amount of air pressure behind the eardrum can help prevent middle ear disease.

ANSWERS: 1-C, 2-A, 3-B, 4-B, 5-A, 6-C, 7-B, 8-B, 9-F, 10-F, 11-T, 12-T, 13-F, 14-F, 15-T

# 2

# EXAMINATION OF THE EAR

# 2 EXAMINATION OF THE EAR

In this section you will learn:

1. How to position children for the examination.
2. How to examine the outer ear and what to look for.
3. How to safely use an otoscope to examine the ear canal and eardrum and what to look for.
4. When to suspect a hearing problem.
5. About professional hearing testing (audiometry).

## *INTRODUCTION*

Because of the limited nature of this book, it is impossible to fully describe the examination of the entire body. However, the importance of a complete examination is not meant to be lessened by this necessary neglect. Frequently, a child who is found to have an ear, nose or throat problem will also have an unrelated problem elsewhere. Furthermore, a number of ear conditions may be part of larger, multisystem diseases. A good example of this is strep throat in which tonsillitis and enlarged lymph glands in the neck might occur along with an ear infection. There is no substitute for a complete examination and no substitute for your physician.

Some children are easier to examine than others but none of them are impossible. With all children you need patience; with most of them you need some help. Always tell children what you are doing and what you expect them to do. Explain everything and be gently reassuring. Talking a lot during the exam keeps little ears busy and establishes a good relationship.

Of course, it's easier to examine a child who is still and cooperative. Although you may not be able to convince them to be cooperative, they can usually be stilled, but do not force the exam on a frightened child. A child old enough to sit quietly is seated in a chair across from the examiner's chair. An active toddler can be held by another adult in the chair, with the child's legs between the helper's legs and the child's upper body and arms held in a loving but firm bearhug. An infant is best examined while lying on its back with someone available to help steady the head. Squirmers can be snuggly wrapped in a large towel to limit arm and leg mobility. Consult your doctor about his or her techniques and other helpful hints. See figures 3, 4 and 5.

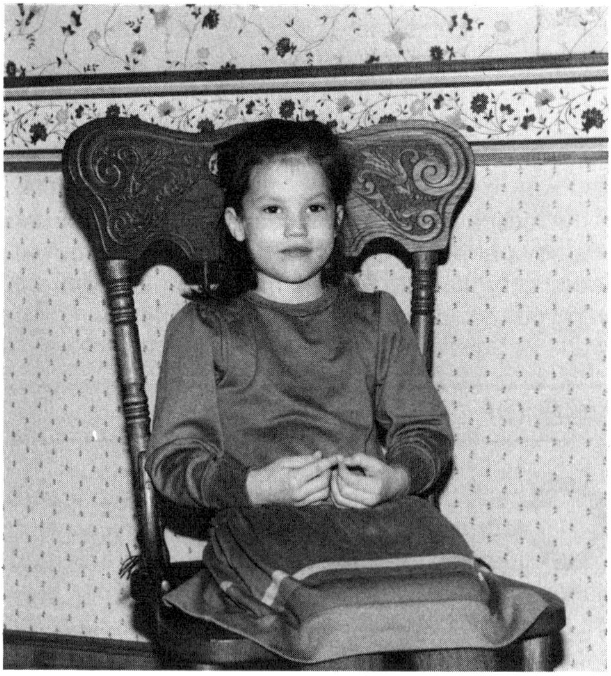

*FIGURE 3*

*Examination of the Cooperative Child*

*The right-handed examiner would be seated to the child's right side. A left-handed examiner would be seated on the opposite side.*

*FIGURE 4*

*Examination of the Not-so-Cooperative Toddler*

*The child is gently but firmly snuggled by the helper, who controls the arms and legs. The child's head is placed against the helper.*

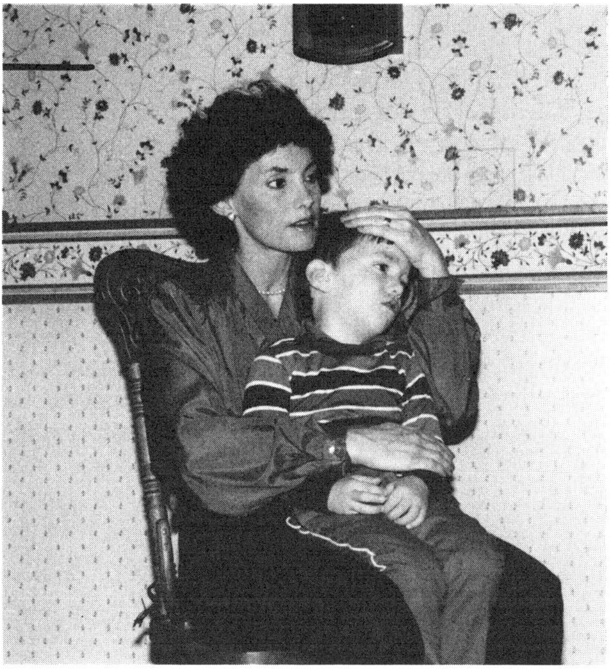

Practice all phases of the exam on your spouse or study partner. It is only with practice that you will become proficient. Seeing many normal ears will help you to recognize the abnormal ones.

## USE OF THE OTOSCOPE

Check the outer ear for tenderness to touch, redness, swelling or evidence of injury. Also feel the area around the ear for enlarged glands (lymph nodes) and note whether or not they are tender. Look at the opening of the ear canal for swelling, redness and drainage. What is the type,

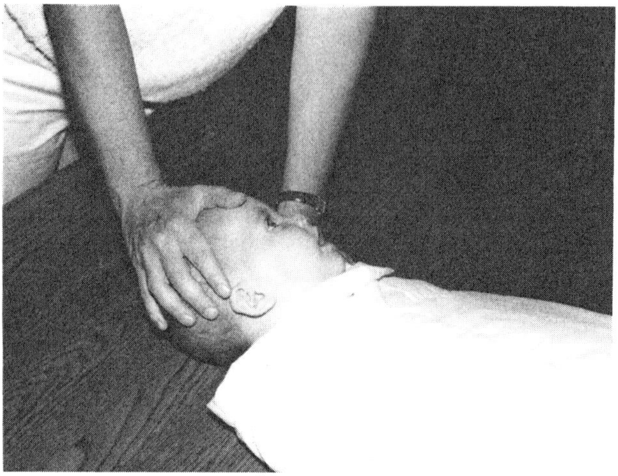

*FIGURE 5*

*Examination of the Infant*

*The infant is wrapped snuggly in a towel or soft blanket to help secure the arms and legs. The helper controls the head.*

color, and amount of drainage? Is there an odor? Does the child have a temperature?

Next, you will use the otoscope to examine the rest of the ear canal and the eardrum. Safe and proper use of this instrument is essential. It is not a toy, so don't let your children play doctor with it. Improperly used, it can cause pain and bleeding and may even rupture the eardrum if inserted too far. You should ask your physician to check you out on the use of the otoscope. Your doctor's help will make both of you more comfortable and confident about what you are doing. Always use fresh batteries; otherwise everything will take on a red hue. Storing the instrument in the refrigerator may help to prolong battery life.

See the otoscope ordering information at the end of the book.

The use of the otoscope is the same, whether the child is seated, being held or wrapped snuggly in a towel for the examination. The hand in which the otoscope is held (always the dominant hand) is braced against the head so that any unexpected motion of the patient causes the examiner's hand and otoscope to move safely with it. The opposite hand is used to help position the child's ear. For the sake of convenience, let's assume that the examiner is right-handed. Left-handed individuals may simply reverse "left" and "right" in the following description. REMEMBER, THE YOUNGER THE CHILD, THE CLOSER THE EARDRUM IS TO THE OUTSIDE AND THE MORE LIKELY IT IS TO BE INJURED. If there is pain at any time, stop the examination and notify your doctor.

First, examine the right ear. Select a clean otoscope tip (speculum) that is no smaller than the ear canal opening and put it on the otoscope. See figure 6. Turn the instrument on. With your free hand, firmly grasp the edge of the outer ear at the ten o'clock position and gently pull it upward, backward and outward at the same time to help straighten the ear canal. Brace your ring finger and little finger against

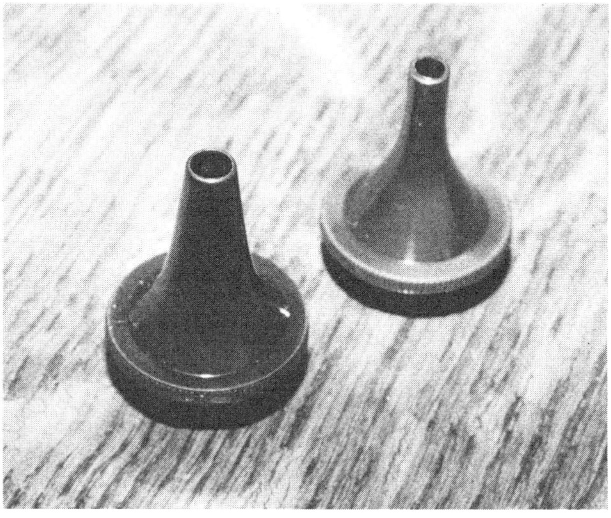

*FIGURE 6*
*Selecting the Correct Size Otoscope Tip*

*Choose a tip that is at least the same size as the opening of the ear canal. Too small a tip may accidentally injure the eardrum or canal.*

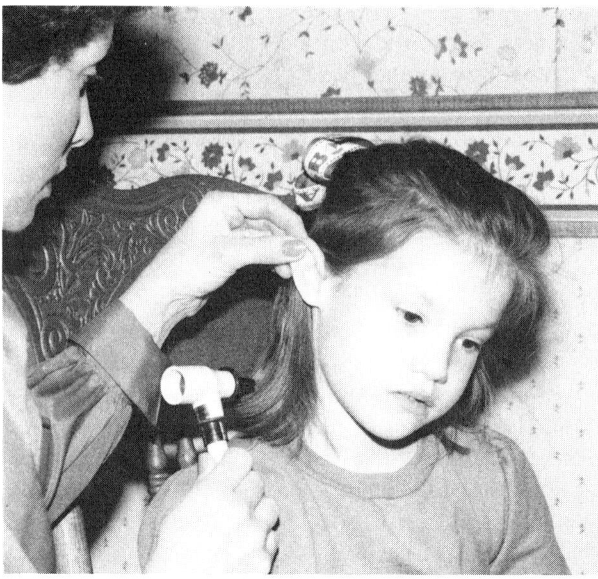

FIGURE 7

*Positioning the Right Ear*

*The right-handed examiner grasps the upper part of the right ear at the 10 o'clock position with the left hand, gently pulling it upward, backward and outward to straighten the ear canal.*

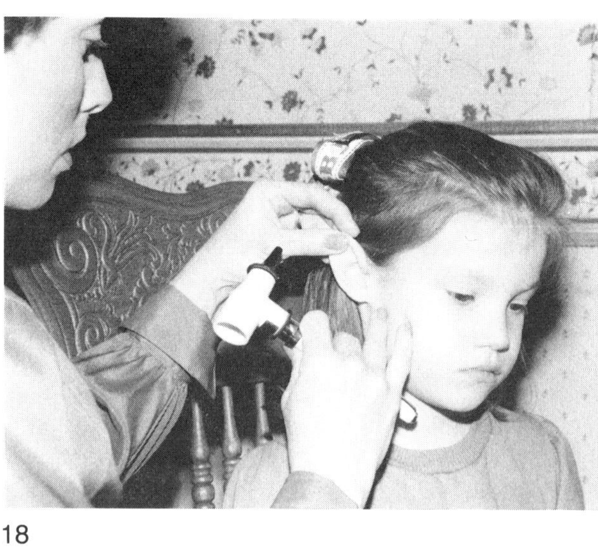

FIGURE 8

*Bracing the Right Hand for Right Ear Examination*

*The fourth and fifth fingers of the right hand are braced against the right cheek. If the child turns his head, the hand and otoscope will safely turn with it.*

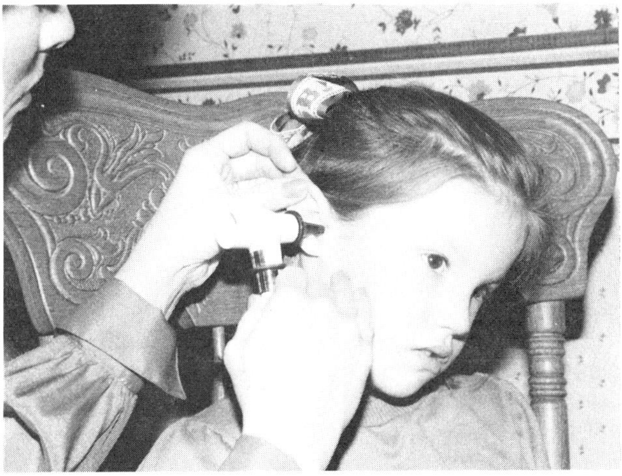

*FIGURE 9*

*Placing the Otoscope at the Right Ear Canal Opening*

*The otoscope is placed AT (not IN) the opening of the ear canal in the right ear. Note that the examiner is not looking through the instrument yet.*

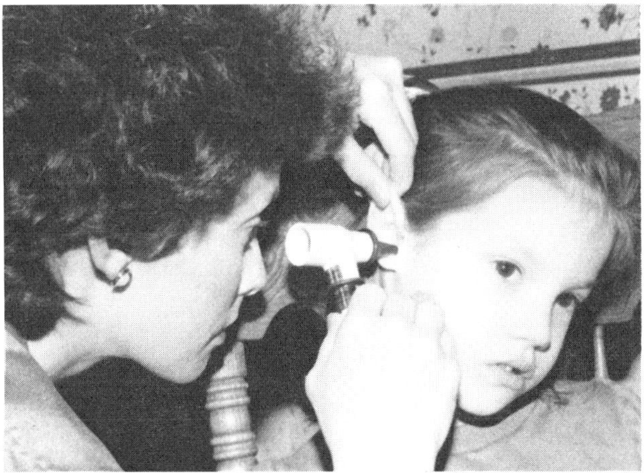

*FIGURE 10*

*Looking Through the Otoscope, Right Ear*

*The examiner is looking through the instrument, first at the canal and then at the eardrum. The head and instrument may be tilted to see all the parts of the canal and eardrum.*

the head to steady the instrument, as if you were steadying a small paint brush. Next, put the tip of the speculum AT (not IN) the opening of the ear canal. Examine the ear canal and eardrum, being careful not to put pressure against the ear with the otoscope. The otoscope may have to be tilted to see all the areas of the eardrum. It's like trying to see all the corners of a room through a keyhole. See figures 7-10. Clean the otoscope tip with alcohol prior to using it on the left ear.

Now check the left ear. The examination is basically the same except for the positioning of the hand holding the ear. For right-handed persons, the left ear is grasped with the free left hand, reaching over the top of the ear and holding it from behind in the 2 o'clock position. Again, it is gently pulled upward, backward and outward at the same time to help straighten the ear canal. See figures 11-14. Don't forget to clean the otoscope tips with alcohol after each use.

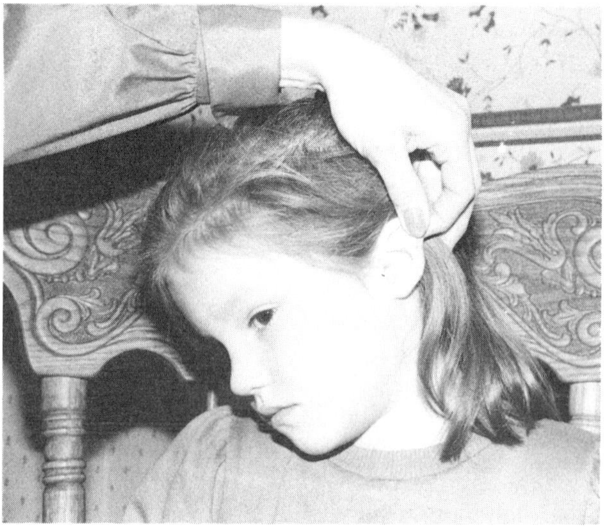

*FIGURE 11*

*Positioning the Left Ear*

*The right-handed examiner grasps the upper part of the left ear at the 2 o'clock position with the left hand, reaching over the top. The ear is gently pulled upward, backward and outward to straighten the ear canal.*

*FIGURE 12*

*Bracing the Right Hand for Left Ear Examination*

*The fourth and fifth fingers of the right hand are braced against the left cheek. If the child turns his head, the hand and otoscope will safely turn with it.*

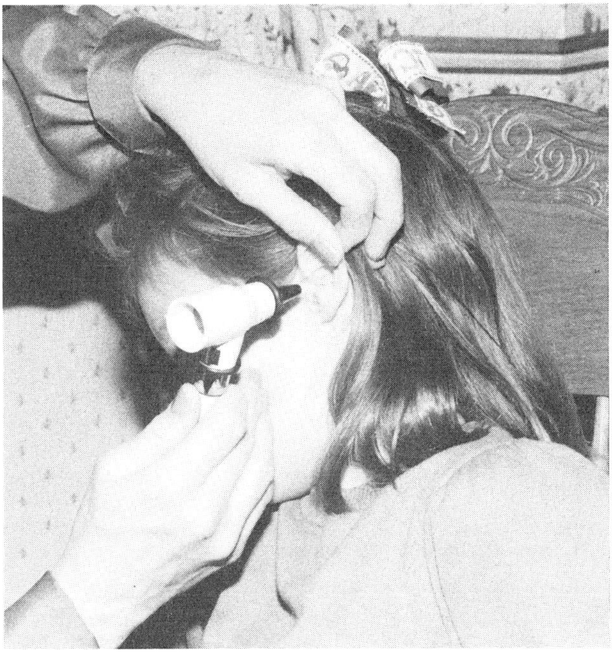

Don't expect to become an expert with the otoscope overnight. It is only with repeated practice and examining many normal ears that an abnormality will be appreciated. Use the color photographs of ears to assist this learning process. Examine your spouse or study partner for practice. Check your children's ears frequently to learn what they normally look like.

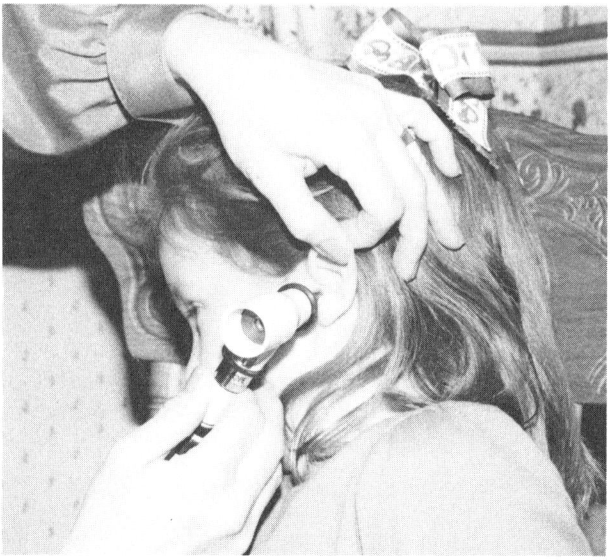

*FIGURE 13*

*Placing the Otoscope at the Left Ear Canal Opening*

*The otoscope is placed AT (not IN) the opening of the ear canal in the left ear. Note that the examiner is not looking through the instrument yet.*

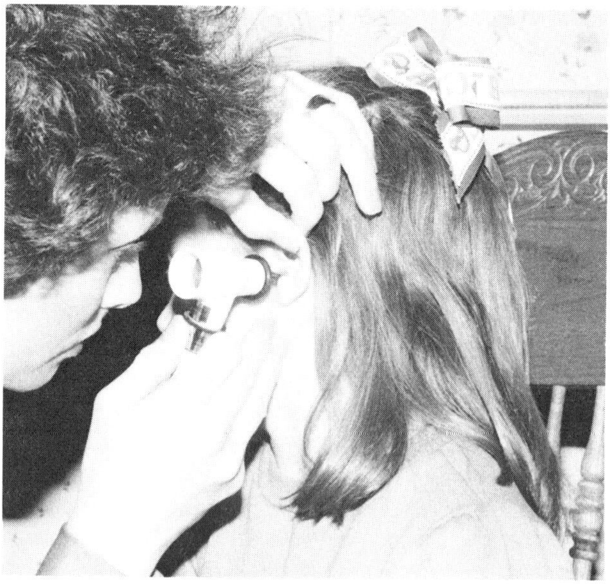

*FIGURE 14*

*Looking Through the Otoscope, Left Ear*

*The examiner is looking through the instrument, first at the canal and then at the eardrum. The head and instrument may be tilted to see all the parts of the canal and eardrum.*

## *WHAT TO LOOK FOR WITH THE OTOSCOPE*

Each external ear canal is examined for swelling, redness, foreign objects, wax, drainage, and evidence of injury (bruises, cuts, or bleeding). Do not attempt to remove wax through the otoscope. Refer to the section on EAR CARE, page 39 for further information about ear wax removal. The eardrums are checked for clarity (semitransparent, like thin wax paper), color (pearly-gray), and position (neither bulging outward nor retracted inward). Is there evidence of middle-ear fluid, such as an air/fluid level or bubbles behind the drum? Is there a hole in the eardrum or drainage from the drum? Make copies of the following EAR EXAM RECORD and use it to note your findings.

## *IS THERE A HEARING PROBLEM?*

In examining the ear, we are not only concerned about its appearance, but also about hearing. A family history of childhood deafness and certain problems in pregnancy, delivery and the neonatal period should alert the physician to evaluate the newborn infant's hearing. If necessary, even day-old babies can have their hearing checked with the use of very sophisticated electronic tests.

Realize that in younger children it is more difficult to evaluate hearing because they are not able to tell you when they hear a sound and may be distracted at the time of the test. It takes a fairly loud sound to get a startle or blinking reaction from a

## EAR EXAM RECORD

Patient: ______________________ Date: __________

History: ______________________________________

_______________________________________________

(Oral/Rectal) Temperature: _____________________

| | RIGHT EAR | LEFT EAR |
|---|---|---|
| External ear | | |
| normal | ☐ | ☐ |
| tender | ☐ | ☐ |
| redness | ☐ | ☐ |
| swelling | ☐ | ☐ |
| Ear canal | | |
| normal | ☐ | ☐ |
| tender | ☐ | ☐ |
| drainage | ☐ | ☐ |
| redness | ☐ | ☐ |
| swelling | ☐ | ☐ |
| foreign body | ☐ | ☐ |
| wax | ☐ | ☐ |
| Eardrum | | |
| normal | ☐ | ☐ |
| can't see | ☐ | ☐ |
| retracted | ☐ | ☐ |
| bulging | ☐ | ☐ |
| red | ☐ | ☐ |
| transparent | ☐ | ☐ |
| dull | ☐ | ☐ |
| air/fluid level | ☐ | ☐ |
| bubbles | ☐ | ☐ |
| cloudy fluid | ☐ | ☐ |
| yellow fluid | ☐ | ☐ |
| perforation | ☐ | ☐ |
| Hearing | | |
| normal | ☐ | ☐ |
| decreased | ☐ | ☐ |
| can't test | ☐ | ☐ |

Impression: ____________________________________

Management: ___________________________________

newborn. A hand clap within two feet of a resting baby should do the job. Six-month-old infants begin to localize a sound by first turning their head in the general direction of the noise. By sixteen months, children will be able to find the source of the sound by head turning and looking in the specific direction. Little bells, squeeky toys or music from a pocket radio should get their attention. A three-year-old should be able to hear a ticking watch. When standing behind a four-year-old, softly ask if he or she would like some ice cream. Of course, no five-year-old will be able to hear you when you tell him to wash hands for dinner if he is watching cartoons, no matter how loudly you yell! Make the test appropriate for the situation.

When testing your child's hearing with various noise-makers, do it in quiet surroundings and don't make the sounds too loud. You're not checking for total deafness, just mild hearing loss!

Too often, misbehavior, speech delays, academic problems and stubbornness are blamed on personality and low intelligence when in fact the child may have a hearing loss limiting his or her abilities. If the progression of hearing loss has been gradual, parents and teachers may not notice any problems until the school nurse does a routine hearing test. If at any time there is a question about whether or not your child has a hearing problem, request a hearing test. Your child's hearing is too valuable to take any chances. Most schools and county health departments are able to do screening tests for hearing loss. Your physician may do tests in his office or know of an ENT specialist or audiologist who does. Your child should be routinely tested every two years, sooner if there is a history of hearing problems.

## *PROFESSIONAL HEARING TESTING (AUDIOMETRY)*

The goal of hearing testing (audiometry) is to determine the extent and site of any hearing loss that may be present. Before reading about hearing testing, please review the material on ANATOMY AND PHYSIOLOGY OF THE EAR, page 3.

There are two basic types of hearing loss: conductive losses and sensorineural ("nerve") losses. Conductive types of losses are mechanical in nature and result from a variety of problems in the external canal, the eardrum or the middle ear space. "Nerve" losses (not due to "nervous" disorders) result from problems in the electrical part of the hearing system, including the hearing organ (cochlea), the hearing nerve and the brain. Conductive losses can generally be corrected; nerve losses can rarely be cured. Some types of diseases cause a combination of hearing losses. Of course, a person could even have two different conditions, each of which may result in a hearing loss, perhaps even of different types in different parts of the ear. For example, a child who has a hearing loss due to a measles infection who gets a middle ear infection with fluid behind the eardrum has both a sensorineural and a conductive hearing loss. See the accompanying chart.

Many different types of hearing tests are available. Which tests are selected depend upon the age and ability of the patient to respond to sounds. Two-year-olds can't be expected to raise their hand when they hear a sound. Also, depending upon the results of a test, a second more advanced test may be helpful to further learn about the type of hearing loss present. The goal of hearing testing is to get the

| | *Conductive* | *Sensorineural* |
|---|---|---|
| Type of Loss: | mechanical | electrical |
| Site of Loss: | canal, drum, middle ear space, middle ear bones | cochlea, hearing nerve, brain |
| Example of Causes: | wax plug<br>foreign body<br>hole in drum<br>middle ear fluid | noise injury<br>measles<br>birth defect<br>brain tumor |
| Curability: | often | rarely |
| Type of Treatment: | medication<br>surgery<br>hearing aid<br>ear cleaning | hearing aid |

*Characteristics of Conductive and Sensorineural Hearing Losses*

most amount of information from the fewest tests (and at the least cost) in order to most accurately answer the questions, "How much loss is present?" and "What is the cause of the loss?" Audiometry is performed by specialists called Audiologists who take extra course work after college to become expert in this important field. Basic screening hearing tests may be performed by nurses or other trained personnel, but for the most accurate results, the services of an audiologist should be sought.

Hearing tests range in complexity from watching a child respond to a hand clap to the computerized technology of brain stem evoked response audiometry. The following is a brief discussion of the basic tests performed.

BEHAVIORAL AUDIOMETRY

Observation of a child's responses to different types of sounds at various loudness levels can be surprisingly accurate in determining hearing ability. An example would be to softly ring a bell behind a two-year-old to see if he or she hears a high-pitched sound. If there is no response, the bell is rung slightly louder until the child turns toward the sound. The softest ring that causes a response is that child's hearing level for that particular tone. See figure 15.

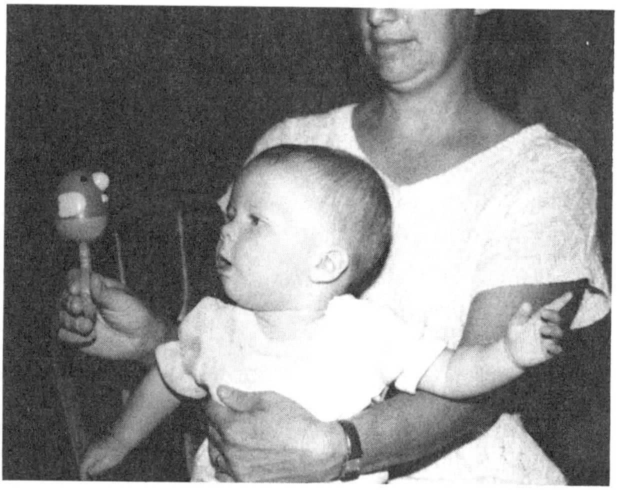

*FIGURE 15*

*Typical Response to Behavioral Test by twelve-month-old*

*The child is turning toward the sound. By sixteen months a child should find the source of the sound with a direct head turn and gaze.*

PURE TONE AUDIOMETRY

In this test the patient is asked to respond when he or she hears tones (like the notes on a piano) at various loudness levels. The results are plotted on an audiogram chart. There are two types of pure tone testing, AIR TESTING and BONE TESTING. With air and bone testing, the part of the hearing system that is responsible for the impairment can be found.

AIR TESTING: The tones are sent to the ear through the air over headphones similar to stereo headphones. The sounds must vibrate the drum, the middle ear bones and then be converted into electrical signals by the hearing organ. These messages are then sent to the brain along the hearing nerve.

BONE TESTING: The tones are sent directly to the hearing organ and on to the brain, bypassing the ear canal, eardrum and middle ear bones. This is done by putting a sound vibrator on the head so that the tones are first heard by the cochlea. Any difference in scores between air and bone testing can be assumed to be the result of a problem in the canal, drum or middle ear. See figure 16.

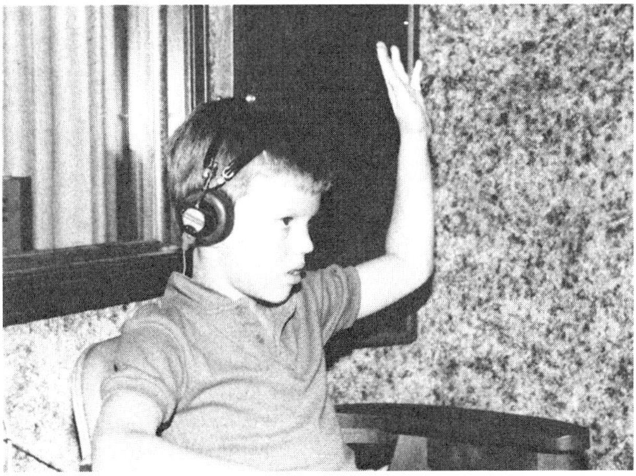

*FIGURE 16*
*Child Undergoing Pure Tone Testing in a Sound Room*

*Older children are able to listen attentively and respond to each sound they hear. A complete hearing test like the one on page 30 can then be performed.*

In charting hearing tests, the loudness of the sound when it was first heard is measured in decibels and the pitch of the note is recorded in vibrations per second. Children older than 12 months should be able to hear a sound of 20 decibels. A 30 decibel hearing loss is enough to interfere with learning. The following chart indicates the decibel loudness of some common sounds.

| | |
|---|---|
| WHISPER AT 3 FEET | 20 DECIBELS |
| WHISPER AT 5 FEET | 30 DECIBELS |
| CONVERSATIONAL SPEECH AT 3 FEET | 60 DECIBELS |
| SHOUTED SPEECH | 90 DECIBELS |
| THUNDER | 90-120 DECIBELS |
| JET ENGINE 100 FEET | 135 DECIBELS |

The audiograms which follow show a child with normal hearing, a child with a conductive hearing loss due to middle ear fluid and a child with a sensory-neural loss due to a measles infection of the inner ear. The symbol "0" is the hearing score for Air Testing and the symbol "<" is the hearing score for Bone Testing. For simplicity, only the right ear is examined.

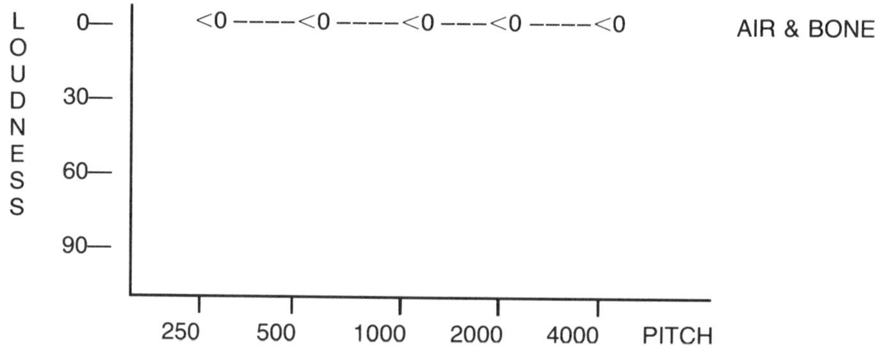


CHILD WITH NORMAL HEARING IN THE RIGHT EAR

*When the tones are presented by air or by bone testing no loss of hearing is found.*

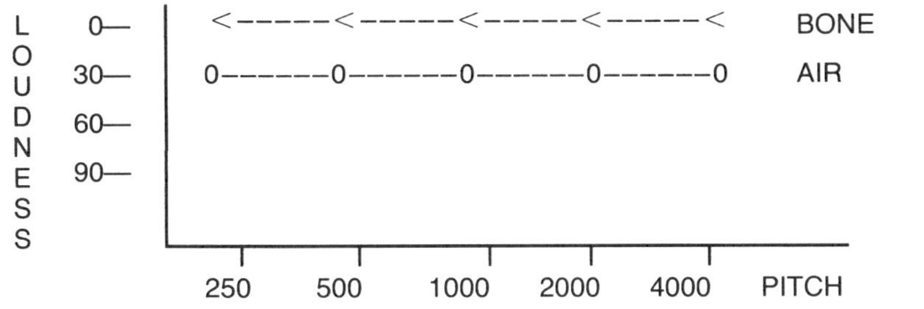


CHILD WITH A CONDUCTIVE LOSS IN THE RIGHT EAR DUE TO FLUID BEHIND THE EARDRUM

*When the tones are presented by air, the middle ear fluid keeps the drum and middle ear bones from properly vibrating. The hearing organ can't hear them until they are 30 decibels loud. When the diseased middle ear system is bypassed with bone testing, the cochlea immediately hears the tones and the child responds.*

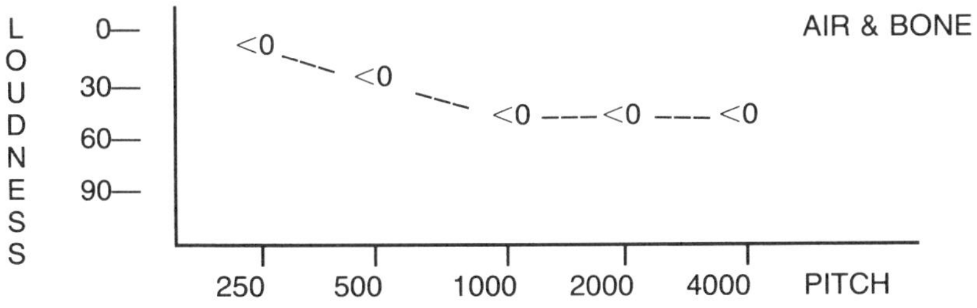


CHILD WITH A NERVE LOSS IN THE LEFT EAR DUE TO MEASLES INFECTION OF THE INNER EAR

*The eardrum and middle ear are not affected by the condition. The diseased hearing organ only allows 30 to 40 decibels of hearing no matter how the sound is sent to the brain, by either air or bone testing.*

## TYMPANOMETRY

This relatively new test checks the functioning of the middle ear system. Results are totally objective: the test can even be performed on sleeping infants. Holes in the eardrum, scars on the drum, vacuum pressures behind the drum, middle ear fluid, plugged ventilation tubes, broken middle ear bones and malfunctioning Eustachian tubes may be suggested by the results of the test. Tympanometry can thus further help to discover the cause of conductive hearing losses.

The technology involved in tympanometry is complicated, but basically the test measures the mobility (compliance) of the eardrum-middle ear system. The results are plotted out and the audiologist or physician interprets the test. This curve has a typical appearance in normal ears, but its shape changes when certain ear prob-

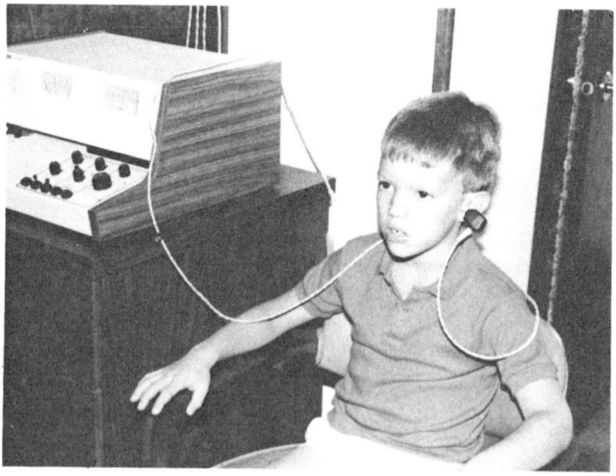

*FIGURE 17*

*Child Undergoing Tympanometry*

*Even a sleeping child can have a tympanogram because the machine does all the work. Tympanograms are useful in screening for middle ear problems but do not actually test the hearing.*

lems occur. Fortunately, the tympanometer machine does all the work while the child simply sits there. Along with the history, physical examination and other hearing tests, a diagnosis is reached. Tympanometry alone is not enough to make a diagnosis. See figure 17.

Because of the simplicity of administering the test it is beginning to be widely used in schools as a screening test for middle ear problems. Tympanograms are often sent home with regular pure tone audiograms and a request from the school nurse to see your child's doctor about a possible ear problem. Also, many pediatricians and family practice specialists now have the ability to do this simple, safe and inexpensive test. There are several examples of tympanogram curves which follow.

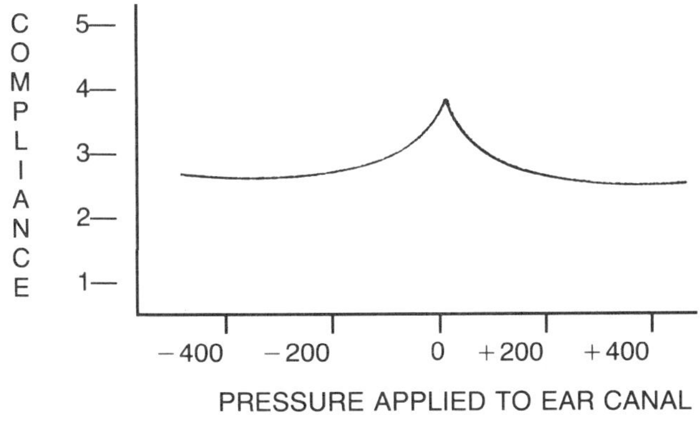


*NORMAL OR "TYPE A" TYMPANOGRAM. Eardrum mobility (compliance ) is at its peak when no pressure changes are applied to the eardrum by the tympanometer.*

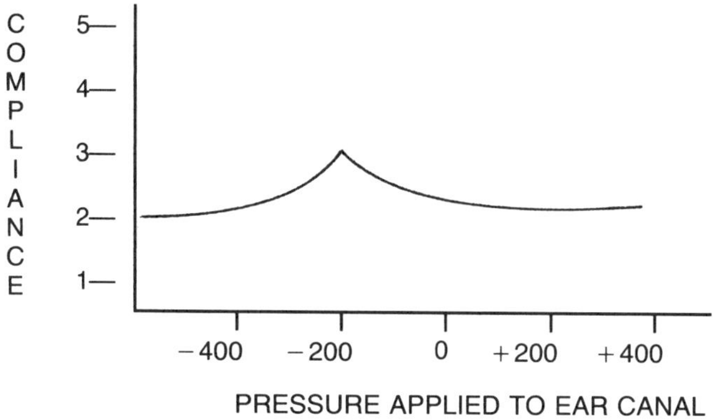


*"TYPE C" TYMPANOGRAM. There is a peak of eardrum mobility shown on the curve but it is only reached when an opposing, vacuum pressure is applied against the eardrum by the tympanometer. This is what happens when there is blockage of the Eustachian tube and the air pressure trapped behind the drum decreases, creating a partial vacuum. Sounds are muffled, but there is no significant hearing loss. If the condition worsens, the peak shifts farther to the left, perhaps to −300.*

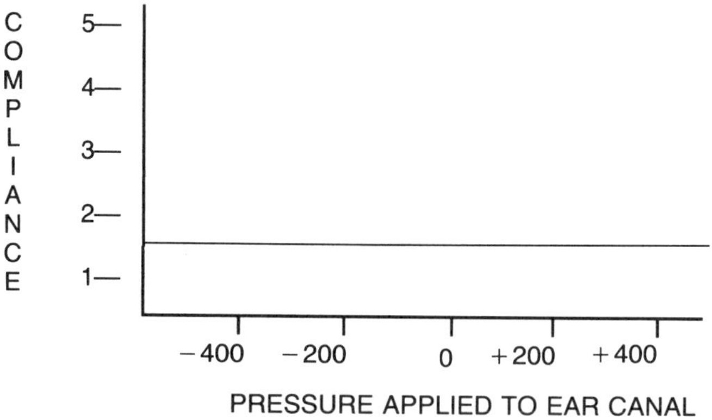


*"TYPE B" TYMPANOGRAM. No matter how much negative or positive pressure is applied, the eardrum and middle ear system show no mobility. There is either an extreme vacuum present or there is fluid behind the eardrum. Sometimes a wax plug in the canal will cause a tympanogram curve to look like this.*

BRAIN STEM EVOKED RESPONSE AUDIOMETRY (BSERA)

A"BSERA" is an extremely sophisticated computerized test which measures the functioning of the various electrical circuits from the hearing organ (cochlea) to the brain. It is most helpful in finding out more about sensorineural (nerve) types of hearing loss and testing small children who are suspected of having hearing loss but who cannot be tested by other means. It is an expensive test and is of no significant risk other than the fact that infants may need to be sedated. Ear specialists will know when a BSERA is needed and who in the area can do it. See figure 18.

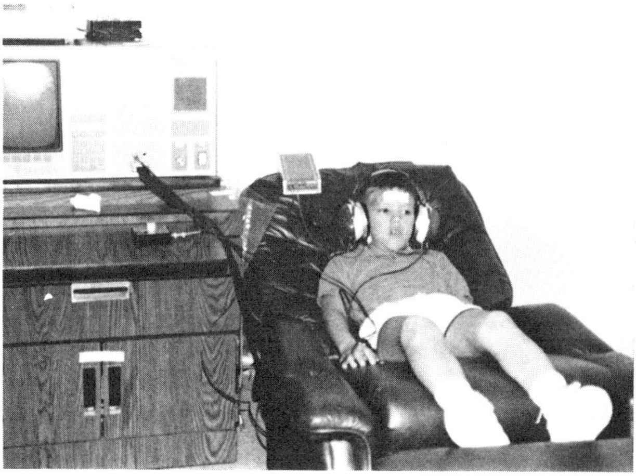

*FIGURE 18*

*Child Undergoing BSERA*

*The brain stem evoked response test is a very sophisticated computerized test. It is most helpful in diagnosing hearing problems in very small children. Because of the cost, it is not routinely performed.*

## FOR REVIEW

I. Match the following (four answers each):
  1. Uncooperative infant examined by right-handed parent, left ear.
  2. Not-so-cooperative toddler examined by right-handed parent, right ear.
  3. Cooperative child examined by left-handed parent, left ear.
  4. Uncooperative Infant examined by left-handed parent, right ear.

    A. Child seated
    B. Child held in chair by helper
    C. Child restrained in blanket, helper holding head
    D. Otoscope held in left hand
    E. Otoscope held in right hand
    F. Left hand braced against cheek
    G. Right hand braced against cheek
    H. Left hand reaches over ear and grasps at 2 o'clock
    I. Right hand reaches over ear and grasps at 10 o'clock
    J. Left hand grasps ear at 10 o'clock
    K. Right hand grasps ear at 2 o'clock

II. True or False
  5. The eardrum is normally pink and dull.
  6. Only a portion of the eardrum is normally seen with the otoscope.
  7. Try to see the eardrum before checking the outer ear for tenderness.
  8. You can't see what is behind the eardrum, only what is on the surface.

9. Newborn babies can always be checked for hearing loss.
10. A type B tympanogram is worse than a type C.
11. A six-month-old should be able to have a pure tone hearing test.
12. Only ear specialists should do and interpret hearing tests.

ANSWERS: 1-C-E-G-H, 2-B-E-G-J, 3-A-D-F-K, 4-C-D-F-I, 5-F, 6-T, 7-F, 8-F, 9-T, 10-T, 11-F, 12-F.

# 3

# EAR CARE

# 3 EAR CARE

Many ear problems can be avoided by understanding how to properly care for the ears. Read this, preach it to your children and then practice what you preach.

## *HOW SHOULD EARS BE CARED FOR ON A DAILY BASIS?*

Ears require little or no care as a matter of routine. They are remarkably self-sufficient! When bathing, the outer ear should be cleaned, but there is no need to try to wash inside the canal with soap and water. This may lead to a higher risk of infection in the external ear. Cotton applicators may be used at the outer part of the canal and to clean the small folds of the ear, but they should not be introduced into the ear canal. This only leads to impaction of any wax which is present, since the swab is about the same size as the canal and acts as a plunger. The canal skin and eardrum can be damaged as well. A small amount of wax is normal and may help prevent ear canal infections. A good rule to follow is to not clean your own ears but to have someone do it for you, cleaning no deeper than they can easily see without extra light. Children follow their parents' example; if they see you cleaning your own ears with a hairpin, they are likely to do the same.

## HOW DO YOU CARE FOR DRY EAR CANALS?

Dry ears are more apt to be a medical problem than those in which extra wax is produced. They are more easily infected and frequently itch. Dry, scaling skin in the ears can even be a sign of a generalized skin problem. Frequent infections of the canal may lead to a dry ear because the wax glands are damaged with the infections. It is easy to see how this can create a vicious cycle. The secret to success for dry ears is to lubricate them with an oily preparation and to avoid getting water in the canals. Sweet oil, mineral oil or baby oil drops are

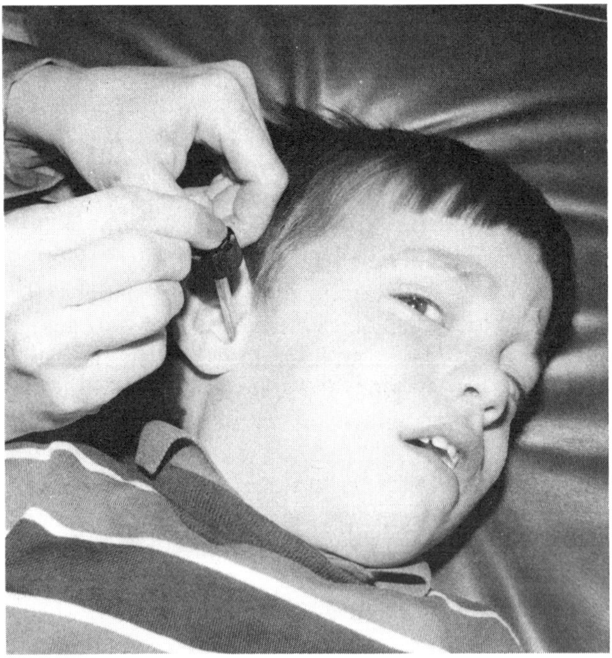

*FIGURE 19*

*Applying Ear Drops to the Right Ear*

FIGURE 20
*Applying Cotton Ball to the Right Ear*

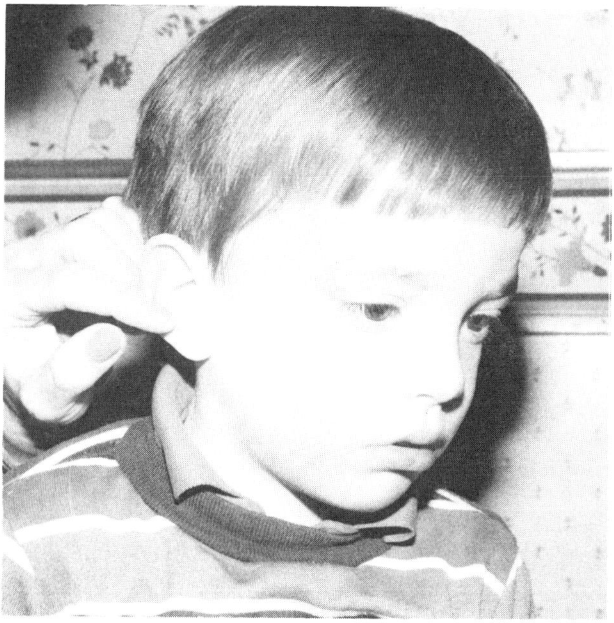

helpful. Apply them only once every week or two. Use five or six drops in each ear and place a large piece of cotton in the outer ear for ten minutes. It is easiest to apply drops with the head turned to one side. Your doctor may recommend a specific medication. See figures 19 and 20.

## *WHAT DO YOU DO ABOUT WAX BUILD-UP*

The first thing to do is to stop using ear swabs if this has been the routine. Chances are good that this alone will solve the problem. If the wax present does not work its way to the outside where it can be easily removed, a few drops of hydrogen peroxide used daily for several days can help to loosen the plug.

There are several commercially available preparations available for cleaning excessive wax from the ear. If the ear is irrigated with an ear syringe, it must not be placed tightly into the canal because it might occlude the canal causing too much pressure and perhaps rupturing the eardrum. Particularly in children, the best advice is to seek professional help if the ear is not easily cleaned.

Very frequently, when examining an ear with an otoscope there will be a small amount of wax in the way, keeping you from seeing as well as you would like. Try to look beyond the wax, as if it was not there. If you have reason to suspect an eardrum perforation, do not use hydrogen peroxide to clean the ear; see your doctor.

## *WHAT SPECIAL CARE NEEDS TO BE GIVEN FOR CHILDREN WHO SWIM?*

This question can be rephrased, "How do you prevent swimmer's ear?" Refer to the discussion of SWIMMER'S EAR (otitis externa) on page 49. Ear plugs are helpful. For frequent swimmers a few drops of mineral oil in the ear prior to swimming helps to keep water from penetrating. After swimming, a twisted end of a facial tissue can be gently worked into the ear without fear of injury in order to help soak up water that may have entered. The use of a commercially available product such as Swim Ear after swimming can help to evaporate any water that has entered the ear canal, and also helps to kill germs. Concentrated ethyl alcohol (grain alcohol from the liquor store is the best) does the same thing.

UNDER NO CIRCUMSTANCES SHOULD ANY DROPS BE PLACED IN AN OPERATED EAR, AN EAR WITH A VENTILATION TUBE PRESENT OR A PERFORATION (EITHER KNOWN OR SUSPECTED) WITHOUT FIRST CONSULTING YOUR DOCTOR. PREPARATIONS CONTAINING ALCOHOL CAN CAUSE PERMANENT DEAFNESS IF THEY ENTER THE MIDDLE EAR SPACE.

The care of ears in which tubes have been placed is discussed in the section on MYRINGOTOMY AND TUBES, page 109.

## *FOR REVIEW*

True or false:

1. Any wax seen in the ear should be removed.
2. If there is not enough ear wax present, an infection of the canal could result.
3. Water irrigations are safe and effective in cleaning wax.
4. Alcohol can cause deafness if it enters the middle ear through a hole or a tube.
5. Teach your children to clean their ears with cotton tip applicators.
6. Mineral oil can be a helpful treatment for dry ears.
7. A painful ear should first be irrigated with hydrogen peroxide.
8. Alcohol can be used to clean drainage from an ear that has been infected.

ANSWERS: 1-F, 2-T, 3-F, 4-T, 5-F, 6-T, 7-F, 8-F.

# 4

# EAR PAIN



---

* indicates the most common causes of ear pain

The following color photographs were provided courtesy of Michael Hawke, M.D. These are examples of right ears. The front is to the right and the back is to the left in each case.

*Normal Eardrum: note the semi-transparent appearance, and the conical shape of the drum. There is a good light reflex in the bottom, front of the drum and the anvil and stirrup are partially seen in the top, back part of the drum in the middle ear space. The blood vessels are a bit more obvious than normal. See page 7.*

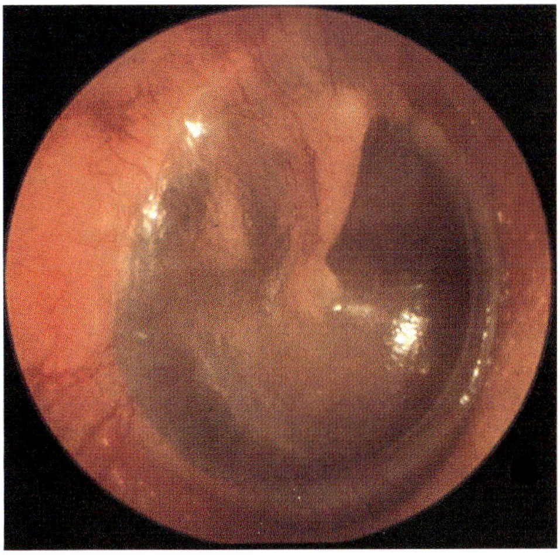

*Color plate 1.*

*External ear canal infection: note the redness and swelling of the outer part of the canal. This ear would be tender to touch. See page 49.*

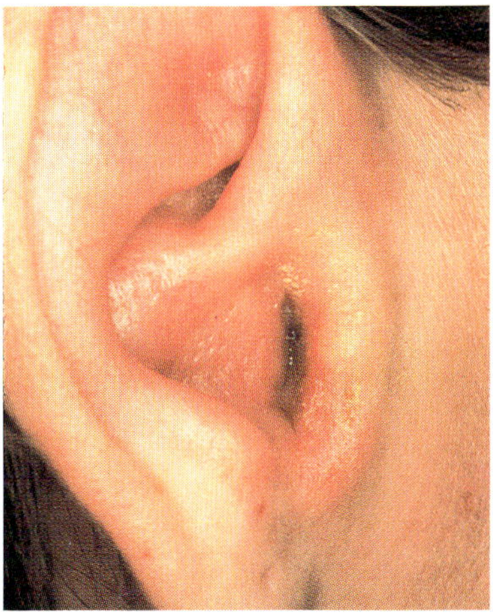

*Color plate 2.*

*Middle ear fluid: note the air bubbles behind the eardrum in the amber-colored fluid. There is no redness. See page 90.*

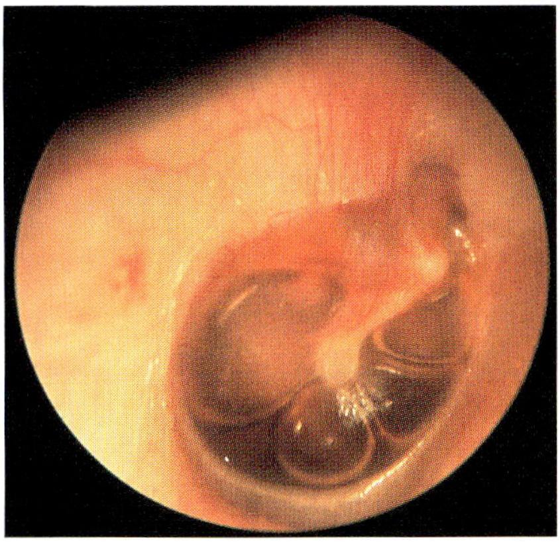

*Color plate 3.*

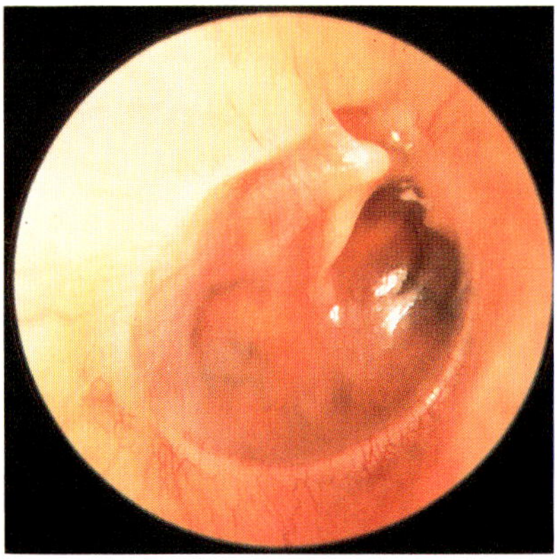

Color plate 4.

*Middle ear fluid with retracted eardrum: note the entire middle ear is filled with a gray-orange fluid. The top, front part of the drum is pulled in toward the middle ear space and the hammer appears especially distinct. See page 90.*

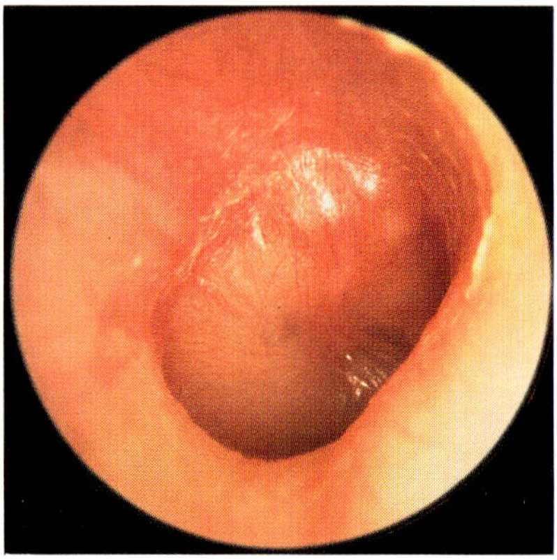

Color plate 5.

*Middle ear infection: note the redness and bulging of the eardrum from the opaque pus behind it. This is a painful ear. See page 55.*

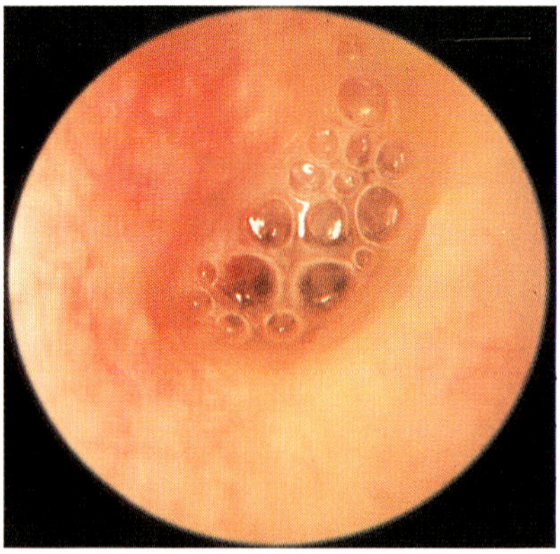

Color plate 6.

*Sudden middle ear infection with perforation and drainage: note the pus in the canal obscuring a view of the eardrum. The bubbles indicate a hole in the eardrum through which air is escaping along with the infection. A painful middle ear infection preceded this drainage. See page 72.*

*Chronic middle ear infection with perforation and drainage: the eardrum is markedly abnormal. There is a pocket of trapped infection and dead skin (cholesteatoma) just above the top of the drum which is the source of chronic drainage and infection. See page 76.*

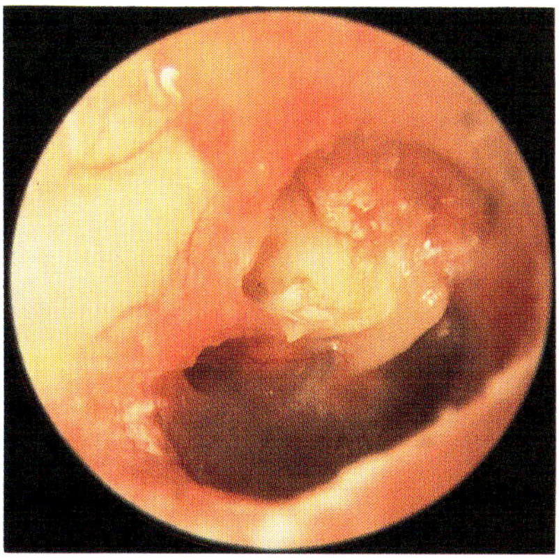

*Color plate 7.*

*Dry perforation of the eardrum: note the normal appearance of the remainder of the eardrum. This small hole occurred from a fall while water-skiing. See page 96.*

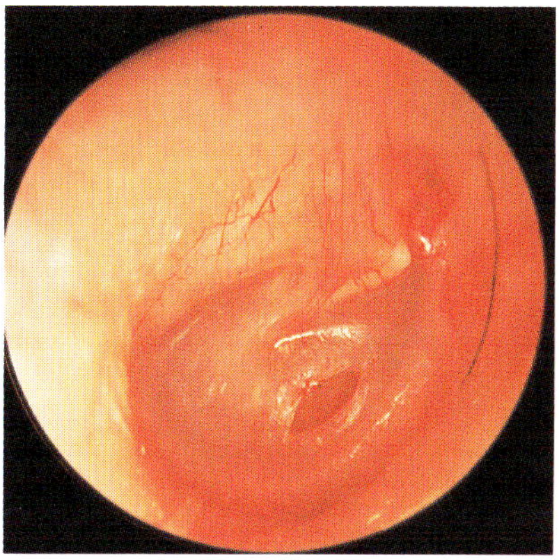

*Color plate 8.*

*Ear tube: the bobbin is in the drum and open. More importantly, the eardrum appears normal. See page 109.*

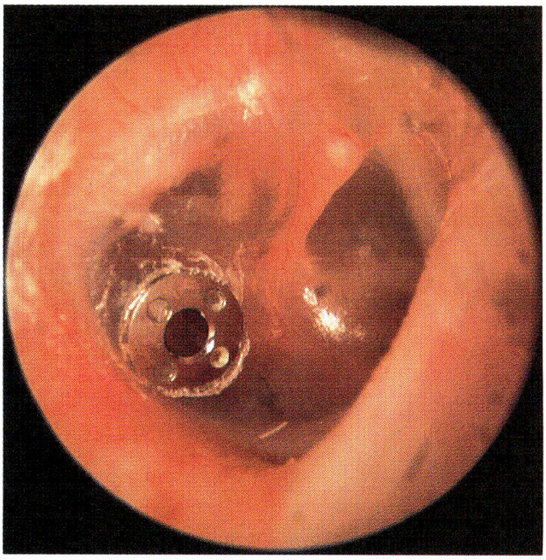

*Color plate 9.*

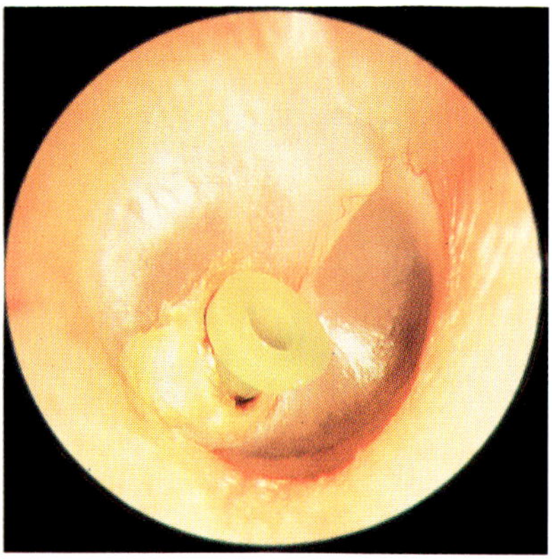

Color plate 10.

*Ear tube coming out: the tube is tilted and there is a build-up of dead skin next to it. This tube will probably come out of the drum in a few weeks. The drum is normal and there is no drainage. See page 109.*

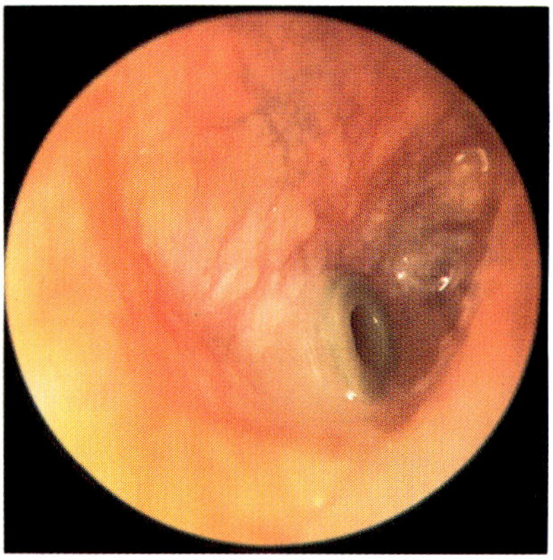

Color plate 11.

*Draining ear tube: the tube is in but there is pus coming through it from the middle ear. The child went swimming. See page 109.*

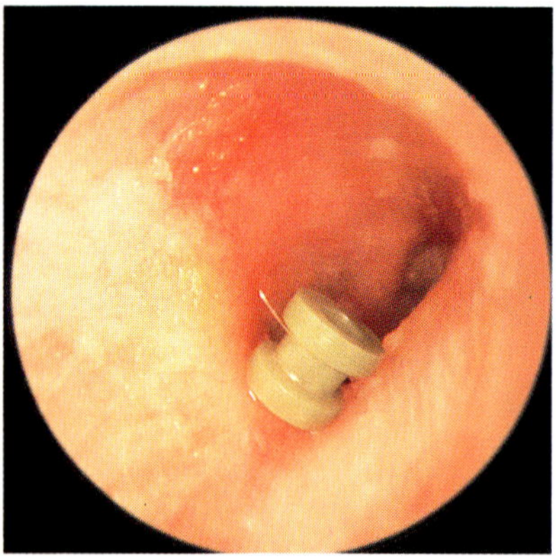

Color plate 12.

*Ear tube in canal: the tube is completely out of the eardrum and lying sideways in the ear canal. The doctor will remove it on the next visit. The drum is not seen. See page 109.*

# 4 EAR PAIN (OTALGIA)

## INTRODUCTION

There are several important features about ear pain which must be understood. The first is that not all ear pain originates in the ear. A number of conditions can cause referred ear pain when there is no ear disease present. This occurs because the nerves which transmit pain signals from the ears also supply other areas in the head and neck. The brain sometimes misinterprets the true source of the pain, blaming the ear.

Another important feature is that the younger the individual, the less he or she is able to accurately communicate specific symptoms. The inability to distinguish pain from pressure, or fullness from hearing loss makes a complete examination necessary. Keep in mind that ear pain is rarely the only symptom present, and that because differences in pain thresholds exist, what is painful to one child is only mildly uncomfortable to another. Furthermore, the absence of pain may be as important a symptom as its presence.

## EXTERNAL EAR INFECTIONS (OTITIS EXTERNA)

Infections of the external ear range from pimples and abscesses to "swimmer's ear," and rarely, life-threatening gangrene. Most cases are readily treated. Most are preventable.

Localized infections, such as pimples and minor abscesses are easily recognized and generally require drainage and antibiotics. Infections of the outer ear involving the cartilage cause the ear to become very swollen and tender. This condition, called chondritis, can result in severe deformity of the ear.

The ear canal is the most common site of external ear infections. Because of the association of this condition with swimming, it is commonly referred to as "swimmer's ear," even though it is often seen in non-swimmers. During hot, humid weather there is sufficient moisture in the air to contribute to infection, not to mention frequent exposure to water with showers and shampoos. It is advisable not to try to wash the ear canal with water because of the risk of introducing bacteria and fungi. Children should be instructed not to place dirty fingers (or anything else) in their ears, and to ask an adult for help if the ears seem to need cleaning. PARENTS MUST SET THE EXAMPLE OF PROPER AND SAFE EAR CARE. For more information see the section on EAR CARE, page 39.

Mild cases of otitis externa can be managed with alcohol or white vinegar ear drops (page 128). More involved or persistent conditions require thorough cleaning of the ear by a physician and the use of oral antibiotics as well as prescription ear drops. Sometimes, a "wick" is placed in the ear to allow the drops to penetrate. CONSULT YOUR PHYSICIAN PRIOR TO USING ANY EAR DROPS IF YOU SUSPECT THERE MIGHT BE A HOLE IN THE EARDRUM OR IF THE EAR DROPS BEING USED CAUSE PAIN.

It is important to realize that a foreign object in the ear canal can result in infection. Middle ear infections draining into the canal through a hole in the eardrum can also appear to be a routine swimmer's ear, when the true problem is a potentially much more serious one. It is a good rule that if the eardrum cannot be seen, due to swelling or drainage, a physician should be consulted.

HISTORY AND SYMPTOMS

Pain is mild to severe, worse lying down.

Hearing is normal unless canal is totally blocked.

Frequently results from getting moisture in ear.

May follow injuries, foreign bodies, or draining middle ear infections.

EXAMINATION

Ear is tender to touch with some watery drainage.

Fever may be present.

The eardrum may be inflamed but hearing is normal because the middle ear space is not involved.

Look for swelling and redness of outer ear and canal.

Local lymph glands are frequently enlarged and tender.

HOME CARE

Carefully clean outer ear and canal (see page 41).

Use ear drops three times daily, changing cotton frequently if eardrum is not perforated. Use ethyl alcohol, Swim Ear, or white vinegar drops (8 drops of 5% white vinegar to 2 teaspoons of tap water).

Use Tylenol for pain and fever.

PROFESSIONAL CARE

Consult doctor if symptoms last more than three days with home treatment.

Consult doctor if there is a history of foreign object in the ear, injury, prior middle ear infection, eardrum perforation, diabetes, or if eardrum cannot be seen.

Antibiotics, professional cleaning, and prescription ear drops may be needed.

PREVENTION

Proper ear care and cleaning (see page 41).

Use preventative ear drops after swimming, such as ethyl alcohol or Swim Ear.

Use of ear plugs for "at risk patients" (frequent prior episodes of external ear infections, diabetics, swimmers).

SEE COLOR PLATE #2

**OTITIS EXTERNA CASE HISTORY**

Josh, age 5, is going through his usual bedtime routine of remembering he forgot to brush his teeth, go to the bathroom and say his prayers. Just as you are about to carry out your threat, he claims to have developed an earache. Likely story. There has been no recent cold and he has not had an ear infection since last Christmas. As you touch his ear he pulls away with a squeal of pain and begins to cry. He does not feel warm and he has been hearing well all day except when you told him to get out of the swimming pool, and of course when you said "lights out."

It's now 1 a.m. and he is still not asleep. Josh feels feverish and says the ear hurts more. An exam with the otoscope shows the canal to be slightly red and swollen in the painful ear. The drum is normal but the otoscope seems to be hurting him. The opposite ear and the rest of the examination is normal.

After five days of white vinegar drops and no swimming he has no pain and his ear exam is normal. He only needed Tylenol for the first day. With the money you saved by not having to take him to the doctor you bought him a new swimming suit and a set of ear plugs.

# *MIDDLE EAR INFLAMMATORY DISEASES*

Without a doubt, the most important topics of this book are the inflammatory middle ear diseases, or "otitis media." These disorders are not presented in continuity in this text because each causes a different main symptom. However, it is important to understand the interrelations of the middle ear diseases. Refer to figure 21 frequently as you read.

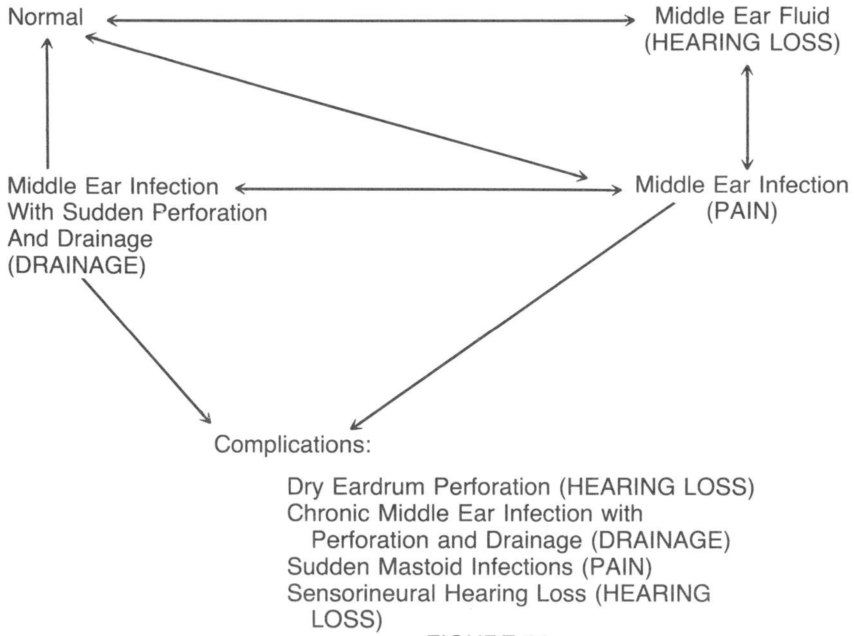


*FIGURE 21*

*The Relationships Between the Middle Ear Inflammatory Diseases*

*Arrows indicate that one condition may lead to another. The major symptom that each condition causes is noted in parentheses.*

The term "otitis media" simply means middle ear inflammation (irritation) and does not always imply the presence of an active infection with bacteria. Middle ear fluid and life-threatening mastoiditis are both examples of "otitis media." Obviously, better descriptive terms are needed to help categorize each condition. They are:

SEROUS OTITIS MEDIA: fluid behind the eardrum

PURULENT OTITIS MEDIA: middle ear infection with pus trapped behind the eardrum.

ACUTE OTITIS MEDIA WITH PERFORATION AND DRAINAGE: A middle ear infection in which the eardrum suddenly ruptures and pus drains out.

CHRONIC OTITIS MEDIA WITH PERFORATION AND DRAINAGE: A middle ear infection in which there has been a longstanding hole of the eardrum that drains pus from time to time.

MASTOIDITIS: infection of the mastoid air cells behind the ear in the mastoid bone, which are connected to the middle ear space.

By definition, an acute condition is one which has occurred suddenly, and a chronic condition is one which has been present for two months or longer. A recurrent condition is one which returns after it has resolved completely.

The key to understanding "otitis media" is the fact that one disease may lead to another more serious one or regress to a milder, less serious one. Don't expect to become a master in understanding the subtleties of all these disorders. That is why there are family physicians, pediatricians and ENT specialists. See color plates 3, 4, 5, 6 and 7.

## *MIDDLE EAR FLUID (SEROUS OTITIS MEDIA)*

This very common condition may precede or follow a painful middle ear infection and is mentioned here for that reason. It is not painful and the usual presenting symptom is hearing loss. See page 90 for a complete discussion of middle ear fluid. Figure 21 on page 53 will help to clarify the important relationships between the various forms of middle ear disease.

## *MIDDLE EAR INFECTIONS (PURULENT OTITIS MEDIA)*

Bacterial infections of the middle ear are quite common in childhood, probably because of the immature structure and functioning of the Eustachian tube connecting the middle ear space to the nose. Also important is the high incidence of upper respiratory infections and allergies in children. It recently has been noted that children of smoking parents have a higher likelihood of developing middle ear infections than others. The disease is also more common in homes that rely on wood heat during the winter months because of the volatilized hydrocarbons in the air. Bottle-feeding infants on their backs may allow milk or formula to directly enter the middle ear. This is possibly a cause of recurrent ear infections.

There is a peak incidence of purulent otitis media between 6 months and 24 months of age, with a gradual decrease in frequency until school age (5-6 years) when exposure to other sick children begins. The condition is markedly less common after the age of 7 years. Nearly 70 percent of all children will have at least one middle ear infection prior to their second birthday.

The symptoms of a middle ear infection are pain without tenderness to touch, fullness and roaring in the ear, hearing loss with the sensation of "being in a barrel," and sometimes balance disturbance (dizziness). The pain is deep, sharp, severe, and may be relieved with elevation of the head. This gives parents the unmistaken impression that the child seems to improve while being held, but as soon as he or she is returned to bed, the pain resumes. Nighttime seems to be the favorite time for pain to begin, when doctors are not readily available, medications are not to be found, tempers are short and everyone needs rest. Infants will not, of course, complain of hearing loss, but may tug at the involved ear(s), even before the pain starts. Because there may have been a preceding episode of middle ear fluid, a dramatic change in hearing may not be noticed when the actual infection starts.

Children with middle ear infections generally have a fever, although this may not be the case in infants less than two years of age. Examination of the ear with a middle ear infection shows a normal canal, decreased hearing and no tenderness to movement of the outer ear, as is the case with infections of the canal. The eardrum is variable in appearance, depending upon the stage of the disease at the time, and whether or not the eardrum has ruptured. Initially, the drum may only show an increase in its blood supply. As infection progresses behind the eardrum it causes the membrane to bulge. By this time the entire eardrum is very red. Cessation of pain in middle ear infections, may be an even more important symptom than its presence, because it may signal rupture of the eardrum with the release of pus into the external canal. The condition now becomes "ACUTE OTITIS MEDIA WITH PERFORATION AND DRAINAGE" (see page 72). With rupture of the drum, blood and pus are seen in the canal, often obscuring the view through the otoscope. As the infection resolves, with treatment, the eardrum begins to return to normal and symptoms disappear.

Home management of middle ear infections is discussed in the accompanying outline. The goal of home care is to relieve pain and attempt to establish drainage of the infection through the Eustachian tube. Physician management is required IN ALL CASES, although your doctor may be comfortable in prescribing antibiotics over the phone. Immediate evaluation is needed for persistant fever, severe headache or stiffness of the neck, dizziness, double vision, or if you are not sure about the diagnosis or the response to treatment. With appropriate treatment, most children are improved within 24 hours, although the appearance of the drum may remain abnormal for several days. Standard antibiotic treatment is for seven to ten days. See the Appendix, page 128.

There are several things that can happen other than complete recovery. First, fluid may persist behind the eardrum (up to 3 weeks is not uncommon), which causes persistent hearing loss and may lead to another infection. (See SEROUS OTITIS MEDIA, page 90). Second, the perforation of the drum (if it did happen to rupture) may not heal, leaving a hole in the drum and causing hearing loss. For more information about DRY PERFORATIONS, see page 96. Such a perforated eardrum may drain off and on, a condition known as CHRONIC OTITIS MEDIA WITH PERFORATION AND DRAINAGE (see page 76). Extension of the infection can even result in MASTOIDITIS (see page 62), meningitis, permanent deafness and paralysis of the face. Any suspected complication of a middle ear infection should be promptly reported to your physician.

Persistent or recurrent infections may require a detailed evaluation for underlying problems, as well as surgical drainage of the infection. The section on MYRINGOTOMY AND TUBE INSERTION, page 107, further discusses this increasingly common surgery for ear infections. Recurrent infections can sometimes be controlled with a preventative course of antibiotics (called chemoprophylaxis) in which a lower dose of antibiotic is given for a prolonged period of time. These options should be discussed in detail with your physician if your child has recurrent or persistent ear infections.

HISTORY AND SYMPTOMS

Deep pain which is relieved somewhat with elevating the head.

Hearing loss or fullness with roaring is usually noted by older children.

Infants are fussy at night, lose appetite and tug ears.

Frequently associated with colds, allergies and sore throats.

EXAMINATION

Fever is usually present in children older than two.

Appearance of eardrum depends upon stage of infection: dilated blood vessels on drum in early stages, cloudy middle ear fluid, red bulging drum later, blood and pus drain from ear if drum perforates.

Mild to moderate hearing loss is usually present.

Ear canal is normal and there is no pain with movement of the outer ear.

HOME CARE

Relieve pain and fever with Tylenol.

Use decongestant nose drops to help internal drainage.

Elevate head and apply warm heating pad.

Use warm ear drops (Auralgan, sweet oil) to ease the pain if there is no drainage or perforated drum.

PROFESSIONAL CARE

Consult doctor for antibiotics and follow-up exam.

A prolonged course of preventative antibiotics may be prescribed for children with recurrent ear infections.

Eardrum may need to be lanced in some cases.

Ear tube insertion may be needed for recurrent or persistant infections (see page 110).

Emergency care is needed for persistent fever or pain, severe headache, facial paralysis, dizziness or stiff neck.

PREVENTION

Early treatment of colds, sinus infection and allergy.

Avoid forceful nose blowing during colds.

Do not bottle feed babies on their backs.

Parents should not smoke if children are otitis-prone.

Surgical management of associated tonsil and adenoidal disease is sometimes needed.

SEE COLOR PLATE #5.

## MIDDLE EAR INFECTION

## CASE HISTORY I

Sonya, age 7, has had a cold for the past week and the secretions have become yellowish in color. She had been doing well until tonight when she woke up with an earache in the left ear. She has had several infections in the past but none since last year. You have not noticed any recent hearing loss but she did bring home a note from the teacher stating she has not been following instructions this week.

After a dose of Tylenol she is again resting, only to wake up at 3 a.m. with severe pain. Her temperature is 100°. The outer ear is normal and not tender to touch. The canal has some wax in it but you are able to see around it well enough to catch a glimpse of the eardrum. It is very red. No bleeding or drainage can be seen. The right ear is normal except for a yellowish discoloration of the drum. There is a lot of yellow mucous in her nose which is draining down the back of her throat. The tonsils were removed two years ago for recurrent strep tonsillitis.

You call your doctor in the morning and he can see you at the hospital on his morning rounds. He congratulates you for an accurate diagnosis: an acute, left middle ear infection and fluid behind the right eardrum. After a 10-day course of antibiotics, a follow-up visit shows Sonya's ears to be normal.

## MIDDLE EAR INFECTION

## CASE HISTORY II

Dennis, age 5 has had middle ear infections each winter for the past three years. He averages four episodes each year. This year appears to be no exception, even though he did very well all summer and fall. In fact, his hearing was normal just three weeks ago on a school audiogram. He has always managed to get over each infection completely. When you examined him with the otoscope last Saturday night the drum was normal. Tonight he is complaining again with earache and fever.

An examination confirms your suspicions. He has a left middle ear infection and the right eardrum seems retracted and dull. His hearing is down in the left ear but he can hear a watch tick on the right. After calling your doctor you begin Dennis on a 10-day course of antibiotics. A week later, the ears are again normal. Your doctor suggests keeping Dennis on antibiotics for the remaining two months of winter. You are told that if this fails to keep him from having infections during that time, he will probably have to have tubes inserted in his ears. The antibiotic is given at one half the usual daily dosage and only once a day.

## *MIDDLE EAR INFECTION WITH SUDDEN PERFORATION AND DRAINAGE (ACUTE OTITIS MEDIA WITH PERFORATION AND DRAINAGE)*

As pressure from pus behind the eardrum builds during a painful middle ear infection, the eardrum may tear, releasing the infection into the external ear canal. As drainage occurs, pressure is relieved and pain subsides. This condition is discussed in depth in the section on EAR DRAINAGE, page 72. The figure on page 53 will clarify the important relationships between the various forms of middle ear inflammatory diseases.

## *INFECTION OF THE MASTOID AIR SPACES (MASTOIDITIS)*

The honeycombed network of air pockets in the mastoid bone behind the ear are connected to the middle ear space and are sometimes involved in middle ear infection as a result of direct extension of the disease. Mild, unnoticed mastoiditis probably occurs each time there is a middle ear infection. Serious cases are unusual today because of early recognition and treatment of middle ear disease. In spite of this, many parents are concerned about the possibility of mastoiditis. There are two types of mastoid disease, the sudden episode (acute mastoiditis) and the long-standing condition (chronic mastoiditis). The most prominent symptom of the acute form is pain, and so, acute mastoiditis is of concern in this chapter. Chronic mastoiditis, on the other hand is characterized more by the symptom of drainage and is discussed on page 76. Both are serious conditions requiring professional care.

Symptoms of acute mastoiditis are pain and perhaps swelling and tenderness behind the ear over the mastoid bone during the course of a middle ear infection. Fever and hearing loss may be present as well. A soft swelling behind the ear causing it to bulge forward probably indicates an abscess. The canal may appear swollen and there is evidence of middle ear infection. Facial paralysis, dizziness, meningitis, brain abscess can result from mastoid infections, but are rare. Obviously if mastoiditis is suspected, immediate evaluation, preferably by an ENT specialist, is warranted. Treatment consists of drainage of the middle ear, antibiotics and sometimes surgery. X-rays of the ear are helpful in discovering the extent of the disease.

## *FOREIGN OBJECTS IN THE EAR*

Children, much more commonly than adults, are seen for foreign objects or "bodies" in the ear. Recognition of the foreign body as the cause of a painful or draining ear and its careful removal are the points to be emphasized. DO NOT ATTEMPT TO REMOVE FOREIGN OBJECTS IN THE EAR. If the object is pushed farther into the canal it only makes it that much more difficult to remove. It is best to leave foreign objects to the care of a physician.

Most, but not all foreign objects in the ear cause pain either initially or eventually, while a few may result in painless hearing loss from blockage of the canal or drainage due to infection or bleeding. Every ear specialist can recall children in whom a foreign body in the ear was discovered on a routine examination, with no symptoms present at all.

Examination of the ear will show the object unless there is so much swelling and drainagae that it is obscured, the ear seemingly involved with an external canal infection. Blood may be present from injury to the canal or the eardrum. Often children are reluctant to be examined for fear of punishment for putting something in their ear. Always check the other ear and the nose as well.

Some objects are more troublesome than others. Vegetable material such as beans tend to cause more local swelling, pain, and infection and should be removed as soon as possible. Solid materials need not be removed immediately unless there is pain or bleeding. On the other hand, foreign objects must never be left to "work their way out."

Insects in the ear present an interesting problem because they are often mistaken for an ear infection due to the extreme pain and anxiety they cause. Clues that this may be an insect are the suddenness of the symptoms and the loud noises they cause in the ear. They must obviously be removed, but can be killed or at least immobilized by putting any oily substance in the ear canal. Attempts to coax the insect out in a dark room with a flashlight are not worthwhile.

## *EAR INJURIES*

Injuries to the ear are best categorized by the part of the ear involved: the ear itself (pinna), and external ear canal, the eardrum and middle ear space, and the inner ear. Most ear injuries require a physician examination because of the risk of infection and hearing loss.

The pinna is susceptible to injuries from blunt trauma, extremes of temperature, and lacerations, not only because of its location but also due to the fact that the underlying cartilage skeleton of the ear has a poor blood supply. A relatively mild blunt injury to the outer ear can cause a blood clot to occur on the cartilage, interferring with the blood flow and ultimately resulting in a deformed ear. This is the cause of "cauliflower ear" in wrestlers and boxers. If a seemingly minor cut becomes infected, the entire ear may become involved, again with the risk of severe deformity.

The most common injuries to the ear occur to the canal and are usually not serious. These generally are due to improper cleaning of the ear or foreign objects. Hearing loss does not occur unless there is damage to the drum as well, but a physician examination is needed if pain, drainage or swelling persist. A small bruise or blood blister of the canal skin is quite painful initially, but can be treated by observation only, unless other symptoms develop.

Injuries to the eardrum can be serious and if suspected, should be evaluated by a physician. A slap on the ear, a fall while water skiing, a foreign object in the ear and careless ear cleaning are the most common causes of non-infectious eardrum perforations. Such an acute rupture of the drum is associated with pain, bloody drainage, hearing loss and ringing in the ear. Most often, the middle ear bones and inner ear are spared from damage and the perforation heals within a matter of days. The examination will usually show the site and extent of the injury. Antibiotics may be prescribed if there has been contamination with water or dirt, but ear drops are to be avoided if possible. Sometimes a paper patch is placed over the hole by the doctor to aid in healing. For larger perforations, or if injury to the middle ear bones is suspected, surgery is needed. If the hole does not heal, or if hearing loss persists when it does heal, consultation with an ear specialist is advisable.

Inner ear injuries are usually caused from major head trauma, such as a fall or automobile accident, or from a deep penetrating injury through the canal. These individuals may have bloody drainage from the ear, a perforated eardrum, and obvious external signs of injury, such as bruising and swelling behind the ear over the mastoid bone. Other neurological signs and symptoms such as loss of consciousness, paralysis of the face, etc. are indicative of the severe nature of the injury. Emergency medical management is needed in all cases. Attempts to clean blood from the canal to allow a better view can introduce germs and must be avoided.

Loud noises can cause ear pain but are most important in that they can cause hearing loss, usually by damaging the delicate inner ear. Such noise trauma to the ear is discussed in the section on HEARING LOSS, page 99.

## *REFERRED EAR PAIN*

These conditions represent a few of the many causes of ear pain not due to primary ear disease. Referred ear pain occurs because the nerves which transmit pain signals from the ear also supply other areas in the head and neck.

Tonsillitis and Pharyngitis
Lymph gland infections
Sinusitis
Dental disorders

## FOR REVIEW

I. Match the following (six answers each):

1. External ear canal infection
2. Middle ear infection
3. Middle ear infection with sudden perforation and drainage

    A. Fever sometimes present
    B. Fever usually present
    C. Fever subsides
    D. Hole in eardrum
    E. Caused by water in the ear
    F. Follows colds and middle ear fluid
    G. Normal canal
    H. Drainage present
    I. Canal swollen
    J. Red eardrum
    K. Try home care
    L. Notify your physician
    M. Tender outer ear
    N. Hearing loss usually present

II. True or False

4. Middle ear infections result from getting water in the ear.
5. Foreign objects in the ear may cause canal infections.
6. Once an eardrum is perforated, it won't heal.
7. Bad teeth cause ear infection.

8. Tonsillitis can cause ear infections.
9. Swimmer's ear may spread to the middle ear and cause mastoiditis.
10. Drainage from a middle ear infection can cause a canal infection.

ANSWERS: 1-A-E-H-I-K-M, 2-B-F-G-J-L-N, 3-C-D-H-J-L-N, 4-F, 5-T, 6-F, 7-F, 8-T, 9-F, 10-T

# 5

# EAR DRAINAGE

*INTRODUCTION*

**MIDDLE EAR INFECTION WITH SUDDEN PERFORATION AND DRAINAGE (ACUTE OTITIS MEDIA WITH PERFORATION AND DRAINAGE)*

**MIDDLE EAR INFECTION WITH CHRONIC PERFORATION AND DRAINAGE (CHRONIC OTITIS MEDIA WITH PERFORATION AND DRAINAGE)*

**EAR WAX (CERUMEN)*

**DRAINING VENTILATION TUBES*

*EXTERNAL EAR INFECTION (OTITIS EXTERNA)*

*FOREIGN OBJECTS IN THE EAR*

*EAR INJURIES*

---

* indicates the most common causes of ear drainage

# 5 EAR DRAINAGE

## INTRODUCTION

Ear drainage is a problem common to many ear conditions, but is rarely the only symptom present. In some cases it may be the most obvious problem while in others it is less conspicuous, being overshadowed by pain or hearing loss. This chapter focuses on those conditions in which drainage is the main problem.

The type of drainage present is a clue as to the nature of the disorder. Foul smelling cloudy mucous obviously represents some type of infection. Fresh, bright red blood is easy to recognize, but old blood clots may be difficult to distinguish from dark wax. Blood clots are jelly-like while dark cerumen has a definite waxy consistency. Although the texture, color, and amount of ear wax (cerumen) varies from one individual to the next, it is fairly constant for a given person. Keep in mind that the course of events preceding the onset of drainage, the presence or absence of other symptoms and findings of the examination are helpful in further determining the cause of the drainage. When there is any doubt about the nature of the illness, a physician consultation is in order.

## *MIDDLE EAR INFECTION WITH SUDDEN PERFORATION AND DRAINAGE (ACUTE OTITIS MEDIA WITH SUDDEN PERFORATION AND DRAINAGE)*

As a complication of a middle ear infection, the eardrum may tear and the pus drain out of the ear. In some children this occurs with each middle ear infection. In others, perforation and drainage never occur. It can be alarming to see blood and pus running from an ear, but it may, in fact, indicate that the infection will soon be over. This does not mean that it is desirable for middle ear infections to rupture the eardrum; hopefully early recognition and treatment can keep this from occurring. This condition, although it represents a stage of middle ear infection, is important enough to demand separate discussion. Please review the section on PURULENT OTITIS MEDIA, page 55.

Since nearly all cases of acute otitis media with perforation and drainage follow a painful middle ear infection, it is usually obvious that something is wrong before the drainage is noticed. When the eardrum perforates, pain subsides and the child may seem dramatically better. Hearing may improve as well. An examination of the ear shows bloody mucous and pus in the canal. If the drum can be seen, a small hole may be present through which drainage seems to pulsate. Several things may happen next.

Usually the perforation heals within a few days (assuming the child is under appropriate treatment). At this time you can sometimes see a small scab on the drum where the tear had occurred. If the infection is not controlled, the drum may perforate again. Sometimes the perforation does not heal and the ear keeps draining. This is called CHRONIC MIDDLE EAR INFECTION (CHRONIC OTITIS MEDIA) WITH PERFORATION AND DRAINAGE. It is discussed on page 76. Another possibility is that the perforation may persist without continued drainage. This is discussed in the chapter on HEARING LOSS under the topic of a DRY PERFORATION, page 96. This may obviously result in further infections since the ear is now open to the outside world. See figure 21 on page 53 to better understand the relationships between the various forms of middle ear inflammatory diseases.

In all cases of suspected acute otitis media with perforation and drainage, consult your doctor. The drainage should be carefully cleaned from the outer ear canal as this can lead to infection of the skin and outer ear. After a week or two, a physician should be seen again in order to examine the eardrum and to check the hearing.

HISTORY AND SYMPTOMS

This condition follows a painful middle ear infection (see PURULENT OTITIS MEDIA, page 55).

Pain, fever, and hearing may improve with drainage.

ACUTE OTITIS MEDIA WITH DRAINAGE AND PERFORATION may mimic external ear canal infections if the canal becomes infected.

In some cases, drainage and pain seem to occur at the same time.

EXAMINATION

Bloody pus is present in the canal and there is

some degree of hearing loss.

A perforation may be hard to see due to drainage; it can heal within five days.

A perforation can remain and result in intermittent drainage, a condition called CHRONIC OTITIS MEDIA WITH DRAINAGE AND PERFORATION (see page 76).

A perforation may persist without ever draining, resulting in hearing loss (see DRY PERFORATION, page 96).

HOME CARE

Tylenol for pain and fever.

Do not put drops in ear without consulting your doctor.

Clean any drainage from the ear canal by frequently changing cotton.

Clean dried secretions from the outer ear with cotton-tipped applicators.

PROFESSIONAL CARE

Consult physician for antibiotics and further care.

Persistent drainage may require cultures and ear drops.

Emergency care is needed for severe headaches, persistent fever, seizures, neck stiffness, facial weakness, or if a painless draining ear becomes painful as drainage ceases.

A followup examination needed to check status of drum and hearing.

Drainage lasting longer than eight weeks may indicate CHRONIC OTITIS MEDIA WITH DRAINAGE AND PERFORATION (see page 76).

PREVENTION

Early detection and treatment of ear infections.

SEE COLOR PLATE #6.

## ACUTE OTITIS MEDIA WITH PERFORATION AND DRAINAGE

### CASE HISTORY

Three-year-old Billy has had a cold for four days, but started to complain about pain in his right ear after dinner yesterday. He was up all night (and so were you) with a fever of 102°, pulling at his ear. It is now 8:00 a.m. and he is no longer crying with pain. His temperature is normal (fortunately, since you ran out of Tylenol with the last dose). You notice a small amount of bloody mucous on his pillow. There is more drainage in the outer ear canal but the ear is not tender to touch. After cleaning the ear with sterile cotton you check it with your otoscope and find a reddened eardrum with pus coming from a small hole in the center of it. You call the doctor.

Billy is feeling well on his 10th and final day of antibiotic. An examination of the ear shows a small blood scab in the area of the perforation, but no hole can be seen. There does not appear to be any fluid behind the drum and Billy's hearing seems fine in the right ear, when you whisper "ice cream" with the tip of your finger in his left ear. You make a note in Billy's medical log and plan to have him checked again in three weeks.

## *MIDDLE EAR INFECTION WITH CHRONIC PERFORATION AND DRAINAGE (CHRONIC OTITIS MEDIA WITH PERFORATION AND DRAINAGE)*

In the section on MIDDLE EAR INFECTION WITH SUDDEN PERFORATION AND DRAINAGE (page 72), it was mentioned that if the hole in the eardrum failed to heal and infection either continued or recurred, a chronic (long-term) state resulted. There are several other ways in which a chronic otitis media with perforation and drainage may occur.

In some cases, the ear is contaminated by germs coming in through a dry perforation (usually by getting water in the ear), or infection spreading from the nose or sinuses. In other cases, part of the eardrum may grow into the middle ear space from negative pressure constantly pulling it deeper and deeper. (Picture what would happen if you placed cellophane over a vacuum cleaner nozzle.) These internal pockets may trap skin cells and debris, so that it cannot be shed from the ear in the normal fashion creating a perfect place for bacteria to grow. These pockets of debris are called cholesteatomas and are similar to skin cysts. In the ear there is little room for such growths. Although they are not malignant, they continue to expand, destroying the important delicate structures of the ear and spreading infection. To make matters worse, further complications such as mastoiditis, paralysis of the face, dizziness, meningitis and brain abscess, can result.

This is why surgery is frequently recommended for these chronically infected ears. The major goal of such operations is to control the infection and not necessarily to restore hearing. If a procedure to restore hearing (repairing the eardrum, middle ear bones and middle ear space) can not be done at the same time, a second procedure may be planned.

By definition, an ear in which a ventilation tube has been placed that drains off and on could be said to represent a form of chronic otitis media with drainage and perforation. These ears usually respond nicely to medical management however, and do not require surgery. See the section on MYRINGOTOMY AND TUBES on page 109 for further information.

Chronic middle ear infection with perforation and drainage does not develop overnight. This condition requires expert care, preferably by an ENT specialist. Again, early recognition and management of ear disease is the best prevention.

HISTORY AND SYMPTOMS

Pus drains painlessly off and on from the ear.

Hearing loss of some degree is usually present and may be the only symptom between episodes of drainage.

Pain, dizziness, facial paralysis, and headache are symptoms of further complications.

Similar symptoms may result from an infected ventilation tube. See page 115.

EXAMINATION

Foul smelling mucous and pus is present in the canal.

Perforation of the eardrum is present but might not be seen because of the drainage. Between episodes of drainage it may be the only finding.

Hearing loss is present and there is usually no fever.

A collection of dead skin may form a cyst behind the drum called a cholesteatoma; it has a pearly white appearance.

Any neurological findings such as facial paralysis or headache with nausea and vomiting may indicate a dangerous complication.

Tenderness or swelling behind the ear may indicate a mastoid abscess, in which pain becomes a major symptom (see page 62).

HOME CARE

Home care is not appropriate if this condition is found. An exam by an ENT specialist is needed.

PROFESSIONAL CARE

Prompt medical management needed as well as hearing tests, X-rays, and possibly surgery.

Emergency care needed for any complication or if a painless, draining ear becomes painful and drainage stops.

PREVENTION

Early recognition and treatment of ear disease.

Surgical correction of dry eardrum perforations.

Avoid getting water in an ear with a known perforation or with a ventilation tube present.

SEE COLOR PLATE #7.

## CHRONIC OTITIS MEDIA WITH DRAINAGE AND PERFORATION

### CASE HISTORY

Your eight-year-old niece has come to spend the week while her parents are on vacation. You were told she has "bad ears" and was not to get water in them. Two days later you find her swimming the creek with your own daughter (who shouldn't be in the water either since she still has ventilation tubes in her ears from last winter). As luck would have it, your daughter did not develop drainage. But cousin Carla did; from both ears. She tells you this happens every time she gets water in her ears and that the last time the doctor treated her, he wanted her to see an ENT specialist for surgery. No wonder they didn't take her to the beach.

Carla denies pain or dizziness with the drainage but you noticed when you first met her that she did not seem to hear well. Now her hearing is even worse. There is a large hole in the left eardrum with pus coming through it, and no eardrum is seen on the right side. There appears to be some shiny white material and old wax mixed with pus where the right eardrum should be.

You take her to your ENT specialist the same day. She orders X-rays which show a definite cholesteatoma in the right ear which has dissolved the mastoid bone over the years. She prescribes antibiotics and ear drops after cleaning both ears under the microscope. A return appointment is made for next week to schedule surgery, when Carla's parents return.

## EAR WAX (CERUMEN)

Wax is a natural, valuable product of healthy ears. Too little wax is more apt to cause ear problems than an excess of wax, although millions of people devote time each day trying to get wax out of ears.

Wax is produced in varying quantities, colors and consistency by glands in the outer part of the ear canal. At body temperature, it remains soft, gradually working its way to the outer ear opening, from where it is shed. Rarely, wax will be produced in such quantity that it builds up in the ear and blocks the ear canal. More often, the canal is plugged by attempts to remove wax with improper use of cotton swabs. These applicators are helpful in removing the wax in the outermost, visible part of the canal, but are usually introduced too far into the ear. Particularly in children, the canal is narrow and the swab acts as a plunger, further impacting the wax. As the liquid wax is pushed off the canal wall, it builds up in the canal and dries there. This quickly leads to wax plugs and the incorrect belief that the ears are producing too much wax.

Ear wax has a specific function: to help prevent infections in the external ear. Bacteria do not grow well in wax, which is slightly acidic in nature. Remove this barrier, and the stage is set for an infection. The trauma of vigorous ear cleaning can further damage the skin of the ear canal and invite infection. To make matters worse, some people then wash out the ear with water, making a perfect environment for bacterial or fungal growth. For these reasons some of the worst ear canal infections may occur in individuals most concerned with ear cleaning.

There is no doubt that ears occasionally need to be cleaned. There is no doubt that cotton applicators are of benefit in helping to do this when properly used. There is also no doubt that ears are best left alone to do their own self-protection and self-cleaning if at all possible. Refer to the section on EAR CARE, page 41.

HISTORY AND SYMPTOMS

Occasional drainage of small amounts of waxy substance from the outer ear.

Pain and fever are not present.

Drainage is not continuous and does not have a foul odor.

Hearing loss occurs if wax totally blocks ear canal.

Tinnitus occurs if canal is blocked or if wax presses against the eardrum.

May lead to symptoms of OTITIS EXTERNA if the canal becomes infected, usually from trying to wash out the ears. See page 49.

EXAMINATION

The appearance of wax varies in amount, color and consistancy from one individual to another.

Sometimes only one ear will make an excess of wax.

Tenderness occurs with movement of the outer ear if infection of the ear canal develops.

HOME CARE

See the chapter on EAR CARE, page 41.

Only clean the outer part of the ear with a cotton applicator.

Do not irrigate the ear with water.

Do not try to pull the wax out with a hairpin.

Gentle irrigations with hydrogen peroxide or

other over-the-counter preparations may be done only if there is no perforation of the eardrum. Remember not to occlude the canal with the tip of the ear syringe.

PROFESSIONAL CARE

If there is any difficulty in removing wax, consult your physician.

PREVENTION

See the section on EAR CARE, page 41.

**EAR WAX (CERUMEN)**

**CASE HISTORY**

After his usual 30 minute morning shower, 16-year-old Nathan complains of not being able to hear his stereo in the left ear. He has checked the headphones, the cables and the receiver controls but can't seem to find the problem. He wants to borrow the car to take his system to the shop before school today. He has never had a hearing problem before and in fact never had an ear infection in his life.

You find your otoscope before he finds your keys. The ears are not tender, but the canal on the left side is totally packed with brown, soft wax and there are cotton fibers imbedded in it from the swabs he denies ever using. The right ear is only slightly better, but his hearing there seems normal to both of you. Since he is already late for the bus, you decide to wait until after football practice to irrigate the ears with hydrogen peroxide. After several gentle irrigations, the wax loosens and all is well again.

## *DRAINING VENTILATION TUBES*

Drainage from an ear in which a ventilation tube has been placed is similar in appearance to that occurring with CHRONIC MIDDLE EAR INFECTIONS WITH PERFORATION AND DRAINAGE, page 76. However, it is generally easily treated with medication and does not necessarily mean there has been a complication. If you are evaluating an ear for drainage in which a tube has been placed, refer to the section on MYRINGOTOMY AND TUBE INSERTION, page 115.

## *EXTERNAL EAR CANAL INFECTIONS (OTITIS EXTERNA)*

Drainage is often associated with this condition, but ear pain is usually the most pronounced problem. Otitis externa, also known as "swimmer's ear" is discussed in the section on EAR PAIN, page 49.

## *FOREIGN OBJECTS IN THE EAR*

Damage to the canal or the eardrum from a foreign body can cause bleeding from the ear. If the object remains in the ear, it can lead to infection, with drainage of pus. Since most foreign bodies initially cause pain, this topic is discussed in detail in the section on EAR PAIN, page 63.

## *INJURIES TO THE EAR*

Drainage of blood from an ear may indicate a recent injury. If you suspect there has been an injury to the ear, see the section on EAR PAIN, page 64.

## *FOR REVIEW*

I. True or False

1. A middle ear infection that begins to drain pus through a hole in the eardrum is a dangerous problem that requires immediate physician care.
2. A canal infection may result from a middle ear infection, but only if the eardrum ruptures.
3. A perforated eardrum which drains from time to time may require surgery.
4. Call the doctor now if a painless draining ear becomes painful as drainage ceases.
5. A cholesteatoma is really just a skin cyst in the ear and is not a serious problem.
6. A child with a history of middle ear infections who develops headache, fever and a stiff neck may have meningitis.
7. Whenever possible keep the ear canal totally clean washing it out with soap and water.
8. Cotton tip applicators should only be used to clean the outer, visible part of the ear.
9. Bacteria grow well in ear wax and this leads to canal infections.
10. Even a small amount of ear wax can cause hearing loss if it keeps air from reaching the eardrum.

ANSWERS: 1-F, 2-T, 3-T, 4-T, 5-F, 6-T, 7-F, 8-T, 9-F, 10-T

# 6

# HEARING LOSS

*INTRODUCTION*

**MIDDLE EAR FLUID (SEROUS OTITIS MEDIA)*

**PERFORATION OF THE EARDRUM WITHOUT DRAINAGE*

**SENSORINEURAL HEARING LOSS*

**MIDDLE EAR INFECTION (PURULENT OTITIS MEDIA)*

**WAX BUILD-UP (CERUMEN IMPACTION)*

*MIDDLE EAR INFECTION WITH SUDDEN PERFORATION AND DRAINAGE (ACUTE OTITIS MEDIA WITH PERFORATION AND DRAINAGE)*

*MIDDLE EAR INFECTIION WITH CHRONIC PERFORATION AND DRAINAGE (CHRONIC OTITIS MEDIA WITH PERFORATION AND DRAINAGE)*

---

** indicates the most common causes of hearing loss*

# 6 HEARING LOSS

## *INTRODUCTION*

Hearing problems can range from mild to severe, from temporary to permanent, and from treatable to incurable. Fortunately, most hearing problems of childhood are mild and treatable. You will find in this chapter that many of the same conditions which cause other ear symptoms may also result in hearing loss. If a hearing loss is suspected, consult with your physician or an audiologist (a trained specialist who performs hearing evaluations).

It is important to understand the differences between "mechanical" (conductive) hearing losses and "electrical" (sensorineural) losses. Conductive hearing losses occur in the middle ear, eardrum or external ear. Usually they are curable. Ear wax, a hole in the eardrum, middle ear fluid or a fractured middle ear bone will result in a conductive hearing loss. Sensorineural losses, on the other hand, are due to problems in the hearing organ (cochlea), the hearing nerve which sends signals to the brain, or in the brain itself, where sounds are analyzed and interpreted. This type of hearing loss is not curable as a rule, but hearing aids may help. Measles, loud noises, birth defects and meningitis may result in a sensorineural hearing loss. Take time now to review the sections on ANATOMY AND PHYSIOLOGY OF THE EAR (page 3) and PHYSICAL EXAMINATION OF THE EAR (page 13).

## *MIDDLE EAR FLUID (SEROUS OTITIS MEDIA)*

The most common cause of disability among school-age children is hearing loss due to the collection of fluid behind the eardrums. This is a major educational and economic problem as well. In years past many children were labeled as poor students when in fact they were suffering from a correctable minor illness, serous (meaning "watery") otitis media.

Although we are doing much better at recognizing and caring for these children today, the condition continues to challenge our diagnostic and financial resources. Parents still bring Johnny in by the shirt collar and announce that they are at the office because the school nurse keeps sending home notices about his hearing. "Johnny can hear," they say, "he's just lazy and stubborn and doesn't like his first grade teacher."

A gradually developing hearing loss is difficult to notice, both for children and for their parents. Often, parents will not notice loss significant enough to be interfering with school work. If there are no other symptoms and you find yourself constantly yelling, correcting, reminding, scolding and repeating, you come to the frustrating conclusion that the disorder is between the ears, not in them. But, if an adult suddenly developed that same degree of hearing impairment, you can bet that he or she would be in the Emergency Room within the hour.

How does fluid develop behind the eardrum? A healthy middle ear is dependent upon a properly functioning Eustachian tube, the passageway between the middle ear space and the back part of the nose. The Eustachian tube allows air exchange in the middle ear with swallowing, yawning and chewing. These pressure changes are what we all notice when flying or even in going up and down hills in a car. If the air pressure on the outside of the eardrum (the same as the pressure in the nose and the "outside world") is not equal to the air pressure behind the eardrum in the middle ear space, you experience that familiar feeling of ear stuffiness, muffled sounds and "being in a barrel" when you talk. This is what happens when the Eustachian tube fails to do its job, as it sometimes does with upper respiratory infections, allergies, enlargement of the adenoids and sinus infections. With continued malfunctioning, a vacuum develops behind the eardrum pulling the eardrum inward (retraction) and, for reasons which are still being debated, fluid forms in the air-containing middle ear space. The presence of this fluid (which is not necessarily infected) causes hearing loss because the drum is unable to effectively vibrate the sounds along the middle ear bones into the hearing organ. Put a finger in each ear and you have a pretty good idea how things sound to Johnny, who thinks that this is the way the world really is supposed to be, frustrated mom and dad, included.

There is both good and bad news about serous otitis media. The good news is that probably 80 percent of all cases of middle ear fluid will return to normal on their own in less than two months, during which time Johnny will hopefully be moved to the front of the class. The bad news is twofold. First, the longer the fluid remains behind the eardrum, the thicker it gets. Although decongestants are commonly used to treat this condition in hopes of decreasing the obstruction of the Eustachian tube and speeding recovery, there is no solid evidence so far that they are of any real benefit. Even if the Eustachian tube does finally open up, this rubbery glue may not be able to drain out. The ear may then need to be surgically drained (see MYRINGOTOMY AND TUBES, page 107). Second, this fluid is an excellent breeding ground for bacteria. This is why middle ear fluid is frequently a precursor to a potentially more serious problem, a middle ear infection (see PURULENT OTITIS MEDIA, page 55).

Be suspicious about serous otitis media as a cause of hearing loss if your child has, or is suspected of having allergies, sinus problems, nasal blockage, snoring, frequent tonsillitis or colds. Although most underlying problems are not serious, there are rare cases of leukemia and tumors in the nose or sinuses causing no symptoms other than hearing loss in one ear from middle ear fluid. Any time serous otitis media persists more than two months, a physician should be consulted. See figure 21 on page 53 to better understand the relationships between the various middle ear inflammatory diseases.

HISTORY AND SYMPTOMS

Younger children may voice no complaints with middle ear fluid.

Fluid may precede or follow middle ear infections.

It may occur secondary to upper respiratory infections, allergy, sinusitis, tonsil and adenoid diseases.

If only one ear is involved, the over-all hearing may not be noticeably diminished. Both ears are usually involved and hearing loss is obvious.

If the onset of hearing loss is gradual, children may not notice their problem.

Sensations of fullness, pressure, popping, and

gurgling are common.

Pain is not present and dizziness is rarely a problem.

Speech and language delays or problems in school with grades are common.

Child may be soft-spoken, inattentive and may even have learned to read lips.

Hearing improves when the condition clears, usually within six weeks.

EXAMINATION

A dull, retracted eardrum with amber colored fluid, air/fluid level or bubbles may be seen.

Hearing loss is present in the involved ear(s), enough to interfere with hearing whispered speech.

Fever is not present unless infection occurs.

Look for findings associated with underlying cause of middle ear fluid (allergies, colds, adenoid enlargement and sinus infection).

HOME CARE

Treatment is directed at improving Eustachian tube function in order to allow air to enter the middle ear space and fluid to drain out.

Oral decongestants are appropriate, but of unproven benefit. Most doctors use them.

Oral antihistamines are needed if allergy is suspected.

Nasal decongestant drops are helpful, but use only as directed.

Since this condition may persist up to six weeks after an ear infection, follow-up examination is important.

Self-inflation of the Eustachian tube is helpful in improving the airation of the middle ear. Children can be taught to force air backwards to the middle ear space by blowing air through the nose as they pinch the nostrils together. This should not be done if there is cloudy nasal discharge, since it can be forced to the ear, resulting in infection. Blowing balloons is also a good Eustachian tube exercise.

Teachers should be notified that the child is having a temporary hearing problem and needs to be seated in the front of the class.

PROFESSIONAL CARE

Consult your doctor for pain, fever or dizziness.

Chronic serous otitis media (lasting longer than two months) or recurrent serous otitis media (more than three episodes in six months) should be evaluated for possible myringotomy (draining the ear surgically). Ventilation tubes are sometimes inserted to insure adequate middle ear airation and to restore hearing (see MYRINGOTOMY AND TUBES, page 107).

Therapy directed to allergies, tonsils and adenoids may be needed.

PREVENTION

Early treatment of colds, allergy, and ear infections.

Infants should not be bottle fed while lying on their backs, since the fluids may drain back to the ear.

Close followup exam of middle ear infections to detect residual fluid.

SEE COLOR PLATE #3 and #4.

## MIDDLE EAR FLUID

## CASE HISTORY

You were just commenting to your friends last week how well four-year-old Megan has been. Although she had numerous ear infections in the past, she has not had any problems in over a year. You have been very careful about checking her ears after each infection to make sure her hearing had returned to normal and that there was no remaining middle ear fluid. (Your sister's little girl had to have ventilation tubes inserted in her ears because of recurrent infections.) Today, Megan failed her preschool hearing test.

She seemed to be hearing well at home but had a problem last week not paying attention and was outright defiant at times. But that is expected at this age, right? You practically have to pry her away from the TV set. And she turns up the volume even though she sits just inches away from it. Tonight you examine her ears and find both canals to be clear of any wax buildup which might cause hearing loss. The eardrum on the left is retracted inward and contains a yellowish puddle of fluid. As she moves her head up and down you can see the fluid shift back and forth. The right eardrum is very dull and retracted; you cannot see any fluid, but it does not look right. She cannot hear whispered speech at all. If she is not looking directly at you she is unable to understand much of what you are saying. The rest of her head and neck exam is normal except for the enlarged tonsils and nasal congestion with clear drainage, which she always has.

After calling your pediatrician he recommends starting her on a decongestant and antihistamine medication along with exercises to open the Eustachian tube. After the second week, you realize she is hearing better. Her ears look normal with the otoscope and her tonsils seem to have decreased in size. Your husband agrees. A repeat audiogram with the preschool nurses confirms that she has improved. The doctor then sees her and diagnoses nasal allergies, which you have already suspected. Ear ventilation tubes will not have to be inserted. The tonsils and adenoids can stay, but the cat must go.

## *PERFORATION OF THE EARDRUM WITHOUT DRAINAGE*

A hole in the eardrum can result from many causes, including improper cleaning, infections, explosive noises and ventilation tube insertion. So long as the perforation remains dry, it is of no great threat to a child's health. It does cause varying degrees of hearing loss however, and water must not be allowed to enter the ear. This can create considerable problems during bathing, shampooing and swimming. For these reasons, if dry perforations do not show signs of spontaneous healing, they are often surgically treated. The timing of the operation and the type of surgery recommended depends upon the circumstances of the individual case. Many times, surgery can be avoided with proper ear care and a simple office procedure in which the eardrum is patched with a small piece of paper to encourage healing.

A perforation of the eardrum may drain off and on with colds and sinus problems, but if the drainage lasts more than two days, a consultation with your doctor is in order. Frequent or persistent drainage may be an indication of a complication (see CHRONIC OTITIS MEDIA WITH PERFORATION AND DRAINAGE, page 76). If there has been a recent injury to the ear, see the section INJURIES TO THE EAR, page 64.

DO NOT PUT ANY DROPS IN AN EAR WHEN THERE MIGHT BE A HOLE IN THE EARDRUM WITHOUT CONSULTING YOUR PHYSICIAN.

### HISTORY AND SYMPTOMS

This may occur after a middle ear infection with rupture of the drum if it does not heal and occasionally after ventilation tubes have come out.

Dry perforations may also result from injury to the ear from a foreign object, explosive noises or a slap to the ear.

Sudden perforations of the drum cause ear pain (see EAR PAIN, page 49).

Decreased hearing is the main symptom, but there may be roaring, fullness, occasional mild discomfort, and dizziness as well.

Drainage can occur with a cold or if the ear is contaminatead with water, but drainage is not the main problem and the ear is usually dry.

EXAMINATION

The ear canal is normal and there is usually no drainage.

Eardrum shows a hole which may vary in size from a pin hole to total absence of the drum.

Hearing is decreased in proportion to the size and location of the perforation. Smaller holes may result in no loss of hearing.

HOME CARE

Do not get water in the ear.

Use drops only under the supervision of a physician and only if there is infection.

Do not keep cotton in the ear, allow exposure to air.

PROFESSIONAL CARE

Physician management (preferably by an ENT specialist) is needed.

A hearing evaluation needed to determine type and degree of hearing loss.

Office treatments and/or reconstructive surgery can often heal the perforation and restore hearing.

Many ear surgeons delay reconstructive eardrum surgery until age 10 because of the greater chance of healing as the number of upper respiratory infections decreases.

PREVENTION

Early recognition and treatment of ear infections.

Proper ear care to avoid injury.

SEE COLOR PLATE #8.

**PERFORATION OF THE EARDRUM WITHOUT DRAINAGE**

**CASE HISTORY**

Nancy comes home from her friend's house and casually announces at the table that she cannot hear from the right ear. She discovered this while listening to records with stereo headphones. When you ask her if she had ever noticed it in school, she admits that she failed a hearing test but was afraid to bring the papers home because you would be mad at her. Her grades have been fine and she has not had an ear infection for two years. She denies any other symptoms or any injury to the ear.

Now that you think about it, you have noticed that annoying habit of hers of turning her head sideways when she talks to you (to put her better ear forward, you guess). An exam with the otoscope shows what appears to be a hole in the center of the drum. There is no evidence of drainage or bleeding. She cannot hear a ticking watch in the right ear. The left ear is normal.

The next morning you call your pediatrician who refers you to an ENT specialist. He agrees with your findings and performs an audiogram which shows a 30 decibel loss in the right ear. Apparently, the last ear infection had resulted in a dry perforation of the eardrum. Because Nancy is 8 years old he recommends delaying any formal surgery until age 10. Instead, he patches the eardrum in the office with a small piece of paper after treating the edge of the perforation to encourage healing. After three weeks the perforation is smaller. After two more patchings, the perforation has completely healed, her hearing is normal and she is able to take swimming lessons. Surgery will not be required.

## *SENSORINEURAL HEARING LOSS*

Hearing loss arising from the inner ear, the hearing nerve or the brain is called sensorineural loss. It is "electrical" in nature as compared to the "mechanical" loss resulting from middle ear disease. Sensorineural losses are generally not preventable and not curable. Many causes exist, including hereditary disorders, problems in pregnancy, certain medications, noise injury, meningitis and brain tumors.

It is important to diagnose sensorineural loss as early as possible. Lack of proper speech development and lack of response to environmental sounds are the usual problems noticed by parents. Physician consultation is needed when this type of hearing loss is suspected; no child is "too young" for a hearing evaluation of some kind.

Treatment depends upon the cause and the amount of hearing loss, but medicines and surgery are usually of no benefit. For the few individuals who become totally deaf (especially after having developed speech), a new and promising operation called a cochlear implant offers some help. Hearing aids are needed for significant losses and should be placed as soon as possible. Many larger communities have excellent programs for hearing impaired children and their parents. The goal for hearing rehabilitation should be nothing less than the normalization of speech, hearing and socialization. Today, children who would have been institutionalized in past years are able to succeed in a normal school setting.

### HISTORY AND SYMPTOMS

Causes include jaundice at birth, Rh incompatability, maternal rubella (German measles), meningitis, ear injuries and certain drugs known to be toxic to the ear.

A family history of childhood hearing loss and the presence of any other birth defects makes a newborn more likely to have hearing problems.

Children with hearing loss present from birth may show a decreased response to environmental sounds and poor development of speech skills.

When older children develop hearing loss, they may verbalize a sensation of fullness, pressure, ringing in the ear or difficulty hearing in school.

Dizziness may occasionally accompany sensorineural hearing loss.

Sensorineural loss alone is not painful.

Symptoms of ringing, roaring or "crickets" in the ear (tinnitus) may be present.

## EXAMINATION

Eardrums are normal, unless there is a middle ear condition present as well.

Infants will eventually show delayed speech and language skills if a significant loss is present.

Reactions to obvious noises in the environment may be absent or seen only with very loud sounds.

Variable responses to noises of different types: if the hearing loss is in the high notes, the child may not hear a phone ring but could hear a man's low-pitched voice and respond appropriately.

Look for any change in hearing ability and slowed development of speech.

Review the section on evaluation of hearing in the chapter on PHYSICAL EXAMINATION, page 23.

## HOME CARE

If there is a suspicion of a hearing loss or if any of the above risk factors are present, a hearing evaluation is needed.

## PROFESSIONAL CARE

Children under age five should be seen by an ENT doctor because of the specialized tests required.

Children age five and older can be initially evaluated by a pediatrician, family doctor or audiologist.

Even newborn babies can be tested to determine if there is a hearing loss present; no child is "too young" for a hearing evaluation and rehabilitation.

The goal of hearing rehabilitation is normalization of hearing, speech and socialization as early, as quickly, and as completely as possible.

## PREVENTION

Most cases of sensorineural hearing loss cannot be prevented.

Recognize and treat ear infections early.

Avoid exposure to loud noises and airtight stereo headphones.

Avoid any medication during pregnancy known to cause hearing problems.

Follow your doctor's advice for prenatal care.

Understand the risks of a family history of hearing problems when planning a family.

## SENSORINEURAL HEARING LOSS

## CASE HISTORY

Michelle is 14 months old. She spent her first night away from you at Grandma's. Your mom asks if you have noticed that Michelle does not seem to be saying any words yet. On the way home you admit that you have been secretly concerned about Michelle's hearing. Has she really been sleeping soundly or does she not hear you when you open her door? Then there was the time that Bill dropped the metal bowl behind her on the kitchen floor. You about jumped out of the chair and little Michelle just sat there like nothing happened at all.

The next day, without telling Bill, you take her to the family doctor who looks in her ears and can find nothing except some ear wax which he removes. He suggests you take her to an ENT specialist for an exam if the loss seems to be persisting. By the time you go for the appointment you are absolutely convinced she has a hearing problem. You can repeatedly slam the door of her room, clap your hands and yell her name without the slightest response. But if you touch her when her back is turned she startles. The specialist can find nothing and tells you that she is too young to test for hearing loss.

Not satisfied with this, you wisely seek another opinion and arrangements are made for specialized hearing tests. Although you find that she does have a hearing problem, it is not as bad as you feared. An evaluation for possible causes of the hearing loss and to discover if there are any other abnormalities is negative. She should be able to develop normal speech and language skills and attend regular school. Hearing aids are placed immediately. Your entire life has changed course. So has Michelle's. In six weeks she says her first word, "mama."

## *WAX BUILD-UP (CERUMEN IMPACTION)*

If wax accumulates in the external ear it may keep sound waves from reaching the eardrum, resulting in hearing loss. Wax is produced in the outer part of the canal and gradually works its way to the outer opening. Attempts to clean it with a cotton applicator may result in the wax being pushed back down into the canal, and even up against the eardrum. Only the outer part of the ear should be cleaned. Please refer to the section on EAR CARE, page 41 for further information. Usually, wax problems cause the symptom of drainage; more about ear wax can be found in the section on EAR DRAINAGE, page 80.

## *MIDDLE EAR INFECTION (PURULENT OTITIS MEDIA)*

Sudden infections of the middle ear can result in hearing loss by interfering with the vibration of the eardrum and the middle ear bones. The hearing loss is usually mechanical in nature and is reversible with early diagnosis and treatment. Rarely, this disease can damage the inner ear, causing a sensorineural loss which may be permanent. Pain is the most obvious symptom of purulent otitis media. This condition is discussed in detail in the section on EAR PAIN, page 55.

## *MIDDLE EAR INFECTION WITH SUDDEN PERFORATION AND DRAINAGE (ACUTE OTITIS MEDIA WITH PERFORATION AND DRAINAGE)*

A middle ear infection which causes the eardrum to tear and drainage to occur causes hearing loss in two ways. First, the infected material behind the drum dampens the sound wave vibrations. Second, when the drum perforates, the eardrum does not effectively transmit the sounds to the middle ear because of the hole. Frequently, as the infected material drains out and the tear in the drum begins to seal, hearing may actually improve. This condition should be treated by a physician. Acute otitis media with perforation and drainage is discussed in detail in the chapter on EAR DRAINAGE, page 72 since that is the most obvious problem.

## *MIDDLE EAR INFECTION WITH CHRONIC PERFORATION AND DRAINAGE (CHRONIC OTITIS MEDIA WITH PERFORATION AND DRAINAGE)*

This condition mostly causes the symptom of drainage, although pain, hearing loss, dizziness and other symptoms may occur. It is discussed in detail in the section on EAR DRAINAGE, page 76. See figure 21 on page 53 to understand the important relationships between the various forms of middle ear disease.

## *FOR REVIEW*

I. Matching:

1. Wax plug
2. Hole in eardrum
3. Broken middle ear bone
4. "Electrical" hearing loss
5. Surgically treatable sometimes
6. Often requires hearing aid
7. May result from measles
8. May result from noise exposure
9. "Mechanical" hearing loss
10. Fluid behind the eardrum

A. Sensorineural hearing loss
B. Conductive hearing loss

II. True or False

11. Anything which causes the Eustachian tube to malfunction can cause serous otitis media.
12. Most of the time, middle ear fluid will clear on its own within two weeks.
13. Treatment of middle ear fluid with antihistamines may be helpful when there are allergies.
14. Pain is a common symptom with middle ear fluid.
15. Children with serous otitis media are usually loud-spoken.
16. The typical findings in serous otitis media are a dull eardrum with amber fluid and perhaps a few bubbles behind it.
17. Surgery should not be considered for treating middle ear fluid until it has been present for six months.

18. Perforations of the eardrum sometimes do not cause hearing loss.
19. Surgery should be performed as soon as possible to repair a perforated eardrum.
20. If a child is not beginning to talk by age 3, a hearing loss may be present.
21. Children not yet in school should not use a hearing aid unless they have a profound sensorineural loss.
22. Loud noises will not damage the ear unless there is prolonged exposure.

ANSWERS: 1-B, 2-B, 3-B, 4-A, 5-B, 6-A, 7-A, 8-A, 9-B, 10-B, 11-T, 12-F, 13-T, 14-F, 15-F, 16-T, 17-F, 18-T, 19-F, 20-F, 21-F, 22-F

# 7

# MYRINGOTOMY WITH AND WITHOUT VENTILATION TUBE INSERTION

# 7 MYRINGOTOMY WITH AND WITHOUT VENTILATION TUBE INSERTION

A myringotomy is a procedure in which the eardrum is incised or lanced. Sometimes a small tube is placed in the opening to keep it from healing closed too soon. It can be performed in the office with local or no anesthesia but is also done as an outpatient hospital procedure under a general anesthetic, particularly in small children. Myringotomies are performed in great numbers today, but there is still considerable confusion as to when they should be done. The information to be presented represents the current consensus among most ENT specialists.

## *INDICATIONS FOR MYRINGOTOMY (WITHOUT TUBE INSERTION)*

There are four major reasons for performing a simple myringotomy. First there is the case of the individual who is having severe pain from a sudden middle ear infection (see ACUTE PURULENT OTITIS MEDIA, page 55). Although it is painful to lance the drum, the pain of the infection quickly subsides. This also allows drainage of the infection. The second reason to do a myringotomy is when there is need to perform a culture of the infected material. This may occur when there is failure to respond to the usual treatment, if the child is a newborn, or if the child is apt to have an unusual type of bacteria due to some problem with the child's immune system (for example, if the child has leukemia or has had a kidney transplant). A third reason to perform a simple myringotomy is when there is a complication of middle ear infection such as meningitis or infection of the balance organ. The fourth reason to do a myringotomy without placing a tube is if the condition is expected to clear up quickly afterwards. Middle ear fluid resulting from pressure changes during airplane travel is a good example.

## *INDICATIONS FOR MYRINGOTOMY (WITH VENTILATION TUBE INSERTION)*

*Middle ear fluid of long duration (see SEROUS OTITIS MEDIA, page 90).* If fluid remains behind the eardrum longer than two months, it is reasonable to assume that it will persist unless removed. If the fluid is removed under a general anesthetic, or if the fluid returns after a simple office myringotomy, insertion of a tube is justified.

*Recurrent fluid behind the eardrum (see SEROUS OTITIS MEDIA, page 90).* If a child has three or more episodes of middle ear fluid in a six-month period of time which clear after each episode, a tube insertion may help prevent future recurrences. Adenoidectomy with or without tonsillectomy may be advised in some of these cases as well.

*Recurrent middle ear infections (see PURULENT OTITIS MEDIA, page 55).* When middle ear infections continue to occur once the ears have returned to normal following adequate treatment with antibiotics, the infections are said to be recurrent. In these situations a reasonable alternative is to treat with a long-term course of antibiotics. Treatment may last through the winter months, for example. The antibiotics are given in one half the amount that would normally be used for an acute infection. If this form of management (called chemoprophylaxis) fails to prevent recurrent infections, then a myringotomy and tube insertion is advised.

*Collapse of the eardrum.* With continued negative pressures behind the eardrum due to poor functioning of the Eustachian tube, the drum may be very thin and collapse as it is pulled inward. This may lead to permanent hearing loss and repeated infection. Sometimes the condition can be reversed with the insertion of a ventilation tube. The eardrum may need to be surgically reconstructed at the same time.

## THE OPERATION

In the office, a myringotomy can be performed without benefit of any anesthetic if necessary. One popular type of anesthetic that can be used is called "iontophoresis." The ear is filled with a solution of local anesthetic such as lidocaine. A small electrical charge is applied to the solution from a battery, causing the medication to numb the eardrum. It takes about ten minutes for this anesthesia to work and many children cannot lie still for that long. Also, if there is an acute infection, the technique does not work very well. In older children and young adults, the ear canal can be injected, in much the same way a dentist injects to numb a tooth.

Obviously, a child must be very cooperative to have tube insertion performed in the office. When tubes must be inserted, it is often easier and safer to do it as an outpatient at the hospital under a general anesthetic. Of course, it is also more expensive.

Regardless of the type of anesthesia used, the operation involves cutting a small hole in the ear-

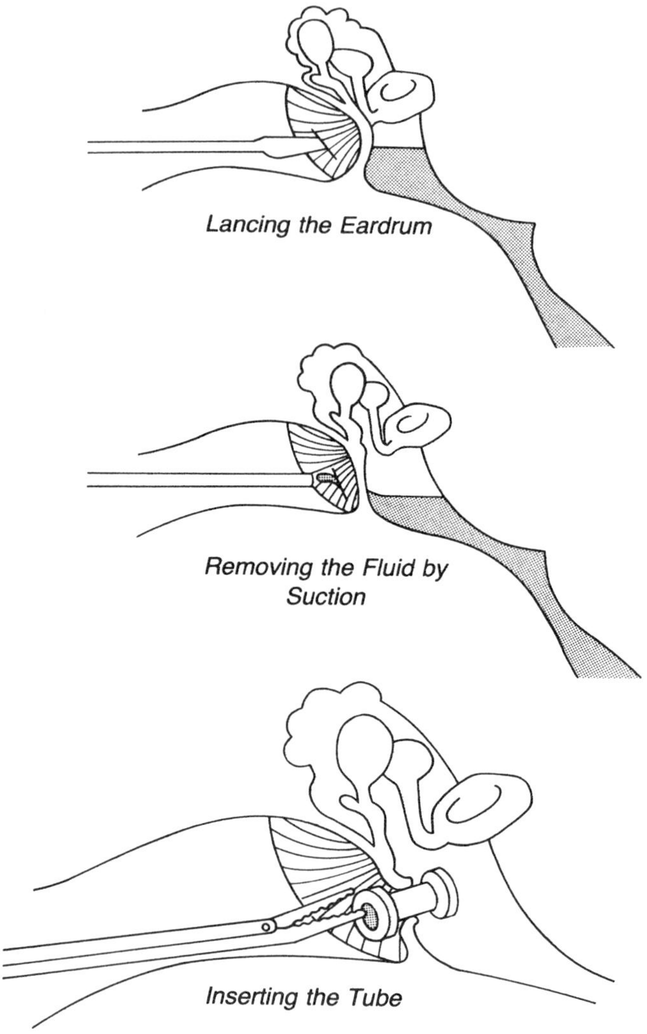


*FIGURE 22*
*The Myringotomy and Tube Insertion Operation. The retracted eardum returns to a normal position when the fluid is removed and the tube is placed.*

*FIGURE 23*

*Some Samples of Ear Ventilation Tubes*

*A. Grommet Tube (6 Months)*
*B. Collar-Button Tube (12 Months)*
*C. Bobbin Tube (12 Months)*
*D. T-Tube (12 Months +)*

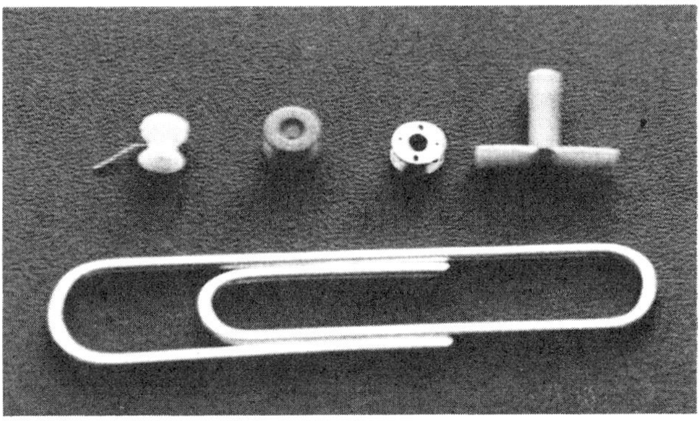

drum and removing the fluid in the middle ear space. See figure 22. If a tube is to be inserted, one is selected that is designed to stay in for the desired length of time. Discuss this with your doctor to decide which type of tube is best under the circumstances. For example, a tube that usually stays in only six months will probably come out when the winter ear infection season starts if it is inserted in April or May. A tube designed to last 12 months may be a better choice. See figure 23.

## FOLLOWING SURGERY

If a general anesthetic is used, the doctor giving it will explain what effects to expect after the operation. These are usually minimal. It is surprising how quickly children wake up, and usually within a few hours they are pretty well back to normal, eating and playing like nothing happened at all. If there is any discomfort, Tylenol in an appropriate dosage may be given. Many children complain for a few days that sounds are too loud if there has been a significant hearing loss prior to surgery. Specific postoperative instructions should be discussed with the surgeon. Usually the child is not allowed to get water in the ears until the tubes are out.

Parents may note some other effects of tube insertion. Children occasionally go through a personality change (for the better) when they are able to hear again. They seem to be in trouble less often, and parents may note that the entire family's life has improved. School grades may suddenly improve. Hyperactive children will sometimes settle down a bit as they are confronted with a new world of auditory stimulation. Fussy babies may sleep better (and so may their parents). Speech may improve in leaps and bounds. Not all of these changes are to be expected in every case of course, but when they do occur they are certainly most welcome!

## *HOME CARE*

If your child has had ventilation tubes placed, you should obtain an otoscope and learn to use it. By examining the ears at home, you can save trips to the doctor, money and your peace of mind. See the ordering information at the end of the book.

Utilizing the principles of examination in Chapter Two, check the ears monthly at least. The important things to note about the ear with a tube are the following:

1. Is the hearing normal?
2. What is the condition of the eardrum and middle ear?
3. Is the tube in or out of the eardrum?
4. Has the tube totally come out of the ear?
5. Is there drainage from the ear?

6. Are the ears still healthy one month after the tubes have come out of the eardrums? Three months? One year?

Many parents become overly concerned about whether or not the tube is still in the drum when the most important considerations are the very reasons for which the tubes were inserted in the first place: hearing and infection. If the child's hearing is normal, but the tube has come out two months before it was "supposed" to come out, that's fine. If the tube is still in the eardrum but fluid has re-accumulated because the tube is plugged with dried secretions, you need to notify your doctor. Tubes may be in place but draining, indicating an infection. If the infection is mild, the drainage may be so slight that it is not noticeable without a careful otoscope examination.

Remember, for the tubes to be functional, they must be in the eardrum and they must be open. A plugged tube or one lying in the canal is not doing its job. If the tube is out of the eardrum or plugged (non-functional) but the hearing is normal and the eardrum is healthy, there is no reason for concern because the Eustachian tube is probably functioning normally. After all, that's the goal of tube insertion. There are some ear specialists who feel that even if a tube is plugged but in the eardrum, air may still be able to get into the middle ear space around the edge of the tube.

Drainage can occur from an ear with a tube in place if water gets in the ear or if the tissues behind the eardrum continue to be a source of infection and mucus production. Any drainage lasting more than two days should be reported to the physician and sooner if there are any associated symptoms of pain, fever or dizziness. Antibiotics and sometimes ear drops are used in these situations. This can be considered a mild form of CHRONIC OTITIS MEDIA WITH DRAINAGE AND PERFORATION, page 76. Do not put any drops in the ear without specific instructions from your doctor.

Keeping water out of ears is not an easy task. If a few drops should enter the ear canal there is no need to panic. If there is a problem, you will notice some drainage of pus from the ear within two or three days (see below). A cotton ball placed in the bowl of the ear and covered with a bit of Vaseline is a pretty good seal for the accidental splash in the bathtub. Nothing can be guaranteed to protect the middle ear from underwater swimming, not even custom made earmolds. There are several soft plugs available that are inexpensive and are better than nothing for the child who is determined to swim. A slight amount of pain occurring off and on is to be expected when the tube begins to come out of the drum. This lasts a few days at the most and may be associated with a small amount of bleeding from the ear. Fever does not occur at this time. Examine the ear to confirm the source of bleeding and call your doctor if you have any questions.

Don't be too eager to celebrate when the tubes have finally come out. The health of the ears is now entirely up to the Eustachian tube. Continue to frequently check the ears, watching for fluid development, hearing loss and infection. Use the principles outlined in this book to guide you. SEE COLOR PLATES 9, 10, 11 and 12.

When the tubes come out, be sure to put them under the pillow for the "Tube Fairy!"

## *PROFESSIONAL CARE*

Contact your doctor for any questions or problems. Your family doctor, pediatrician or ENT specialist will probably want to examine the ears every two or three months after surgery until the tubes have come out and the eardrums have healed. A repeat hearing evaluation is helpful to make sure the hearing has completely recovered. A follow-up ear exam in three to six months is usually recommended after the tube has come out.

# APPENDIX

## MEDICATIONS

*DECONGESTANTS*
*ANTIHISTAMINES*
*FEVER AND PAIN MEDICATIONS*
*NASAL DECONGESTANT SPRAYS AND DROPS*
*SALT WATER NASAL SPRAY AND DROPS*
*EAR PREPARATIONS*
*ANTIBIOTICS*

# APPENDIX

## INTRODUCTION

It is impossible to adequately cover the many excellent over-the-counter (OTC) medications that are available. This chapter presents some of the medications that are commonly used and readily available. The information contained here does not constitute an endorsement of any product over any others. As with all medications OTC preparations should be used only according to the directions on the labels. Obviously, the decision of which (if any) medication to use without the advice of your physician is a personal one for which you alone are responsible. There is a trend toward the use of single-ingredient preparations; some of the medications discussed below were selected for that specific reason. PLEASE KEEP ALL MEDICATIONS OUT OF THE REACH OF CHILDREN.

## DECONGESTANTS

Decongestants are designed to shrink tissue swelling in the nose and sinuses, in order to relieve congestion and promote drainage. Decongestants may help to reduce the stuffiness associated with allergies, but do not interfer with the allergic reaction the way antihistamines do. Sometimes a child's activity level will rise with decongestant use, particularly for the first several dosages. Individuals with high blood pressure, heart problems, diabetes or thyroid disease should not use decongestants except as advised and supervised by a physician. Many OTC nose and sinus decongestant preparations contain antihistamines. Some have cough suppressants, expectorants, aspirin and even caffeine. An excellent single ingredient medication, reasonable in price and pleasant to the taste is Sudafed. It comes in a variety of strengths and forms (liquid and capsule).

SUDAFED SYRUP (30 mg./5ml.)

| | |
|---|---|
| age under 2 years: | consult physician |
| age 2 to 6 years: | ½ teasp. every 4-6 hours, not to exceed 4 doses in 24 hours. |
| age 6 to 12 years: | 1 teasp. every 4-6 hours, not to exceed 4 doses in 24 hours. |

SUDAFED TABLETS (30 mg.)

| | |
|---|---|
| age 6 to 12 years: | 1 tablet every 4-6 hours, not to exceed 4 doses in 24 hours. |
| over 12 years: | 2 Tablets every 4-6 hours, not to exceed 8 tablets in 24 hours. |

Sudafed syrup contains no alcohol and may be stored at room temperature, but protected from light.

## *ANTIHISTAMINES*

This class of medication stops allergic symptoms by blocking the activity of histamines which are released during the allergic reaction. They are often in combination with decongestants and other ingredients. Side effects of antihistamines may include drowsiness, sedation, hyperactivity, nervousness, dry mouth and frequent urination. Antihistamines are most helpful for allergic problems; their use in the common cold and sinusitis may make matters worse, particularly if secretions are thick to begin with. Children on antihistamines should be encouraged to drink liquids. Because of the sedative effect of many types of antihistamines, activities requiring clear thinking and quick reflexes (school work, sports and bike riding) may be affected. Occasionally, children will show excitation as a temporary side effect. Antihistamines should not be used for lower respiratory problems, especially asthma. Overdosage of antihistamines can result in hallucinations, seizures, and death.

Dimetane Elixer is an excellent single-ingredient over-the-counter antihistamine to have on hand. Please note that Dimetane "Decongestant" Elixer also contains a decongestant medication.

DIMETANE ELIXER (2 mg./5 ml.)

age 2-6 years with physician supervision: ½ teasp. every 4-6 hours, not to exceed 6 doses in 24 hours.

age 6-12 years: 1 teasp. every 4-6 hours not to exceed 6 doses in 24 hours.

DIMETANE TABLETS (4 mg)

age 6-12 years: ½ tablet every 4-6 hours, not to exceed 3 tablets in 24 hours.

over age 12 years: 1 tablet every 4-6 hours, not to exceed 6 doses in 24 hours.

Dimetane elixer contains 3% alcohol. Report any suspected side effects to your physician.

## FEVER AND PAIN MEDICATIONS

There are two types of OTC medications that are useful for the relief of pain and fever in children: the salicylates (aspirin) and the acetaminophens (Tylenol, Panadol, Tempra, etc.). Both are essentially equal in effectiveness for the control of pain and fever. For stronger pain medications a physician should be consulted.

Recently there has been some evidence to suggest that there may be a link between the use of aspirin and the development of Reye's syndrome, a devastating neurological illness.

Aspirin can contribute to bleeding problems and so should not be used before or after surgery without

TYLENOL DOSAGE SCHEDULE

THE FOLLOWING DOSAGES MAY BE GIVEN 4 TO 5 TIMES DAILY, BUT NOT TO EXCEED 5 DOSES IN 24 HOURS.

| *Age* | *Infant Drops (80 mg./0.8 ml)* | *Childrens Elixer (160 mg./teasp.)* | *Childrens Chewable Tablets (80 mg.)* |
|---|---|---|---|
| 0-3 mo. | 0.4 ml | | |
| 4-11 mo. | 0.8 ml | ½ teasp. | |
| 12-23 mo. | 1.2 ml | ¾ teasp. | 1½ tabs |
| 2-3 yrs. | 1.6 ml | 1 teasp. | 2 tabs |
| 4-5 yrs. | 2.4 ml | 1½ teasp. | 3 tabs |
| 6-8 yrs. | | 2 teasp. | 4 tabs |
| 9-10 yrs. | | 2½ teasp. | 5 tabs |
| 11-12 yrs. | | 3 teasp. | 6 tabs |
| > 12 yrs. | one or two tablets of regular strength Tylenol every 4 to 6 hours, not to exceed 12 in 24 hours | | |

Consult your physician if fever persists for more than three days or pain for more than five days. Also consult your physician before using Tylenol in children under two years of age.

physician approval. Read the package information carefully prioir to using either aspirin or acetaminophen products. In order to avoid accidental overdosage, be aware that many OTC preparations contain these medications.

The accompanying table shows the appropriate dosages for Tylenol.

## *NASAL DECONGESTANT SPRAYS AND DROPS*

Nasal decongestant sprays and drops are very easy to misuse and abuse. Never use them for more than three days, or they may cause an increase in nasal congestion and discharge. Be sure to select the proper strength of the medication. Sharing nose drops or sprays may result in the spread of infection.

Since the solutions are supplied in generous quantities (more than a three days supply for one person), most of the medicine is wasted and should be discarded. To get around this problem, ask your pharmacist for a clean brown glass dropper bottle. Use the bottle you purchase as a "stock supply," transferring medicine as you need it to the "patient bottle" which can be boiled between usages.

Decongestant nasal drops are useful in relieving the symptom of nasal congestion from the common cold. Symptomatic improvement may be temporarily obtained when used for allergies or sinus infections, but other medications, such as antihistamines or antibiotics may be needed. Neo-Synephrine is widely available in a variety of strengths and in drops or spray.

NEO-SYNEPHRINE (phenylephrine hydrochloride):

age under 2: consult your physician

age 2-6: ⅛%

age over 6: ¼%

Drops are easier to use in children. When applying drops, the child should be lying on his or her back with the head tilted back and toward the side in which the drops are to be placed. Use 2 or 3 drops on each side in this manner. Wait five minutes and repeat for best results. Sprays are used in the upright position, twice on each side.

## *SALT WATER NOSE DROPS*

Many nasal conditions can be helped with the use of a mild salt water (saline) nasal solution in either drop or spray form. During the winter, when the humidity is low indoors from heating, the occasional use of such a solution will help to keep nasal and sinus secretions thin and draining properly. Moisturized nasal membranes can also help prevent the drying and cracking that leads to nosebleeds.

The correct way to make a saline solution so that it is similar in concentration to normal body fluids (and thus does not irritate the nasal membranes) is as follows. In one quart of boiled water dissolve 1½ teaspoons of table salt and allow the solution to cool. This is placed in either a clean dropper bottle or spray atomizer and used as needed, usually 4-5 times daily. The solution should be made fresh each week, because bacteria will begin to grow in it and may cause infection.

Ocean Mist and Ayr Mist and Drops are two salt

water nasal preparations available over-the-counter. Both are excellent and contain preservatives to limit the growth of contaminates, so they have a longer shelf life than the home-made preparations. Do not share these sprays as infection may be spread from one person to another.

## *EAR PREPARATIONS*

No ear drops should be placed in an ear without the direction of a physician if there is a known or even suspected eardrum perforation. Ear wax removal products available include Debrox Drops and the Murine Ear Wax Removal System.

The ears do a very good job of self-cleaning and usually there is no need for the routine use of these preparations (see EAR CARE, page 41). Occasionally, a child will rapidly accumulate wax leading to blockage of the ear canal. In this situation, the drops may be used, following the instructions carefully.

Hydrogen peroxide can be used at home for the removal of accumulated ear wax. It is basically the same active ingredient that is contained in the commercially available products. A few drops in the ear may help to loosen the wax enough that it comes out on its own. Sweet oil, baby oil or mineral oil can help to lubricate a dry ear. A few drops in each ear every week is sufficient.

To help prevent swimmer's ear, mineral oil or sweet oil drops can be applied before swimming and alcohol drops can be used after. DO NOT PUT ALCOHOL IN ANY EAR UNLESS YOU ARE POSITIVE THERE IS NO EARDRUM PERFORATION, AS IRREVERSIBLE DEAFNESS MAY OCCUR. Grain alcohol from the liquor store is highly concentrated and works well to collect and evaporate any water left in the ear canal.

For mild swimmer's ear a solution of water and vinegar can help to eliminate the infection. Add 8 drops of 5% white vinegar to two teaspoons of tap water. This can be used three times daily (see OTITIS EXTERNA, page 49).

There are several antibiotic ear drop preparations available with a prescription. Among them are Cortisporin Otic solution and suspension, Pyocidin-Otic, Coly-Mycin Otic, VoSol and VoSol HC. An ear drop that is helpful for relieving pain from middle ear infections is Auralgan. It does not contain antibiotics. When applying ear drops, use them at body temperature; if they are too hot or too cold, they will be uncomfortable and may cause dizziness.

## *ANTIBIOTICS COMMONLY USED FOR MIDDLE EAR INFECTIONS*

Antibiotics are used for one purpose: to treat bacterial infections. They have no role in the management for viral infections or allergies. Because some bacteria are killed by only certain types of antibiotics, many different drugs have been developed. Some types of bacteria have even started to fight back by making enzymes to counteract the effects of the antibiotics, necessitating stronger and often more expensive medications. The battle is between the bacteria causing the infection and the medication; the body is simply being used to get the drug to the battle zone, whether it is the ear, throat or sinuses.

The key to knowing which antibiotic to select depends on the type(s) of bacteria found in the infection. To determine precisely which bacteria are present a culture can be taken, the germs identified and tested to see what type of antibiotic will do the job. This is called a culture and sensitivity test. It is often impractical to do this "C & S" on ear infections because of the need to lance the eardrum to obtain the sample as well as the expense involved. Furthermore, the test takes several days to perform and treatment is needed now. This means that someone must make a decision about which bacteria are most likely to be the cause of the infection and which antibiotic is most likely to work. Also to be considered are possible side effects, allergic reactions to the medication, the expense and availability of the medication, and the proper dosage. Obviously, selecting an antibiotic requires considerable knowledge and judgement. Antibiotics should be used only under the supervision of your physician.

Middle ear infections require 7 to 10 days of treatment. Ampicillin has been commonly used as a drug of first choice but because of increasing problems with bacterial resistance, many physicians are now initially treating with amoxicillin or the sulfa drugs. Infections not responding can be treated with cefaclor (Ceclor), or amoxicillin with potassium clavulonate (Augmentin). The combination of an erythromycin and sulfa (Pediazole) is also often used for middle ear infections.

Recurring infections can sometimes be controlled with preventative use of an antibiotic. Usually either an amoxicillin or sulfa is used. By giving the medication at one-half the usual total daily dose and administering it once a day, undesirable side effects can be avoided and the medication used for an extended time.

The following chart shows the normal dosages of some of the commonly used antibiotics for treating an active middle ear infection.

Ampicillin (Omnipen, Amcill, Polycillin)
22# 1 teasp (125mg/5ml) every 6 hours
33# 1½ teasp (125mg/5ml) every 6 hours
44# 1 teasp (250mg/5ml) every 6 hours

Amoxicillin (Amoxil, Larotid, Polymox, Trimox, Wymox)
20# 1 teasp (125mg/5ml) every 8 hours
40# 1 teasp (250mg/5ml) every 8 hours

Trimethoprim Sulfa/Sulfamethoxazole (Bactrim, Septra)
20# 1 teasp every 12 hours
30# 1½ teasp every 12 hours
40# 2 teasp every 12 hours

Cefaclor (Ceclor)
20# 1 teasp (125mg/5ml) every 8 hours
40# 1 teasp (250mg/5ml) every 8 hours

Amoxicillin with potassium clavulonate (Augmentin)
20# 1 teasp (125mg/5ml) every 8 hours
40# 1 teasp (250mg/5ml) every 8 hours

Erythromycin/Sulfoxazole (Pediazole)
18# ½ teasp every six hours
35# 1 teasp every six hours
53# 1½ teasp every six hours

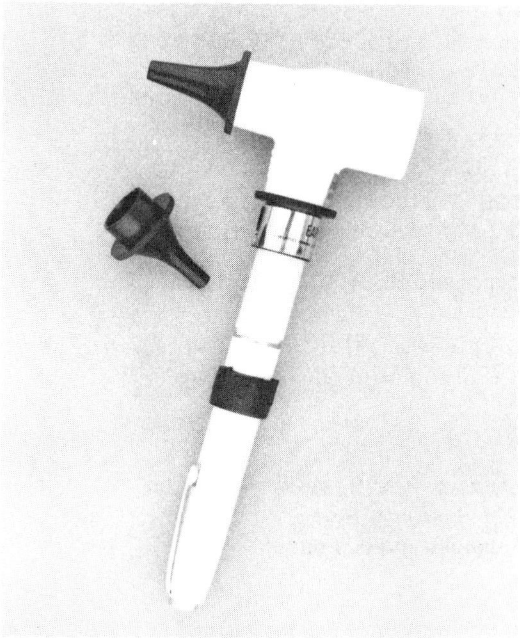

I highly recommend the Earscope by NOTOCO. I have seen many different otoscopes, both professional and economical designs. Without a doubt, the Earscope is the best buy for the dollar. The optics are as good as any professional model I have used. It's what I keep on hand at home for examining my own children.

If you have friends whose children have ear infections or tubes, tell them about The Ear Book and the Earscope. You might even get them a set for a family Christmas gift. Let your doctor know about them too. Discounts are available for orders of six or more.

If you have any comments about this book, please write to me at Lang E.N.T. Publishing, P.O. Box 6846, Jefferson City, MO 65101.

David R. Marty, M.D.

# INDEX

## ORDERING INFORMATION

### The Ear Book

### The Earscope

**TOTAL**

Send me _____ Ear Book(s) @ $16.95 ea. _______

Send me _____ Earscope(s) @ $25.95 each. _______

Missouri residents add 6.225% sales tax. _______

($1.06 for each Ear Book, $1.62 for each Earscope)

Add $1.50 shipping per order _______

TOTAL _____________

Payment enclosed ☐ Visa ☐ MasterCard ☐

Credit Card Account No. ________________

Exp. Date _________

Signature ______________________________

NAME ______________________________

ADDRESS ____________________________

CITY ________________ STATE _____ ZIP _____

Mail to:

Lang E.N.T. Publishing
P.O. Box 6846
Jefferson City, MO 65101

Please allow 6 weeks for delivery.

Phone orders accepted 314-893-5545.

For quantities of 6 or more please inquire about discounts.

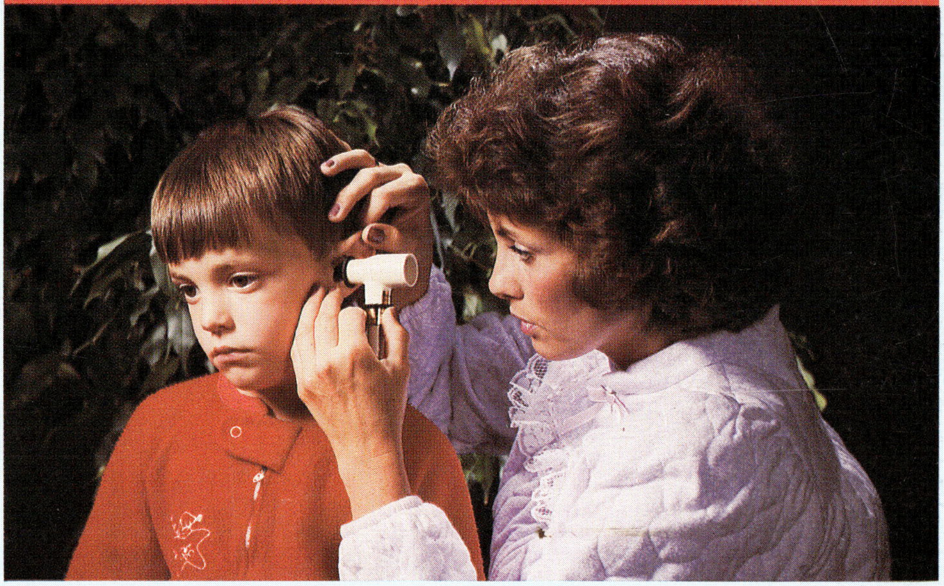

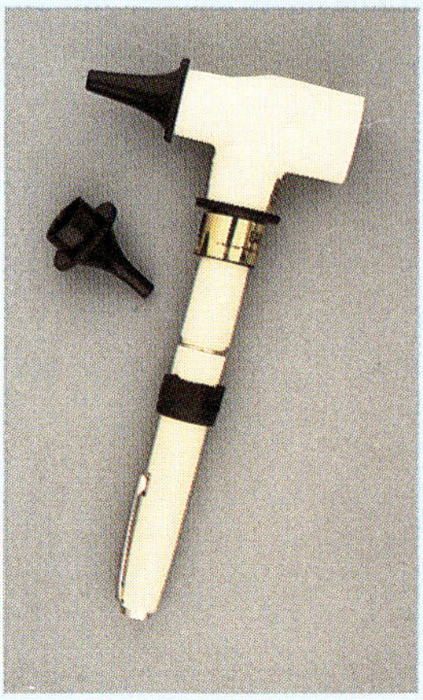

Finally . . .

A book for parents about their children's ear problems:

* How to obtain and safely use an otoscope
* How to recognize and manage common ear disorders
* When to call your doctor
* When your child needs ear tubes

Clearly and concisely written in everyday language
Problem-oriented format
Photographs and illustrations to help your understanding
Color photographs of actual ear disorders
Sample case histories
Self assessment tests
Order forms for otoscopes

The Ear Book is a MUST for any parent whose child has had ear problems. Written by a practicing Ear, Nose and Throat Surgeon (and father of three), this book will save you money, sleep and calls to your doctor. It may even save your child's hearing.

LANG E.N.T. PUBLISHING • JEFFERSON CITY, MO.

ISBN 0-943023-12-2